MIDWIFE CRISIS

From Trust to Trauma
A Midwife's Journey Through a Broken System

Kelli Zakharoff

First published by Ultimate World Publishing 2024
Copyright © 2024 Kelli Zakharoff

ISBN

Paperback: 978-1-923255-28-9
Ebook: 978-1-923255-29-6

Cover art: Melissa La Bozzetta
Layout and typesetting: Ultimate World Publishing
Editor: Marinda Wilkinson

Ultimate World Publishing
Diamond Creek,
Victoria Australia 3089
www.writeabook.com.au

ULTIMATE WORLD
PUBLISHING

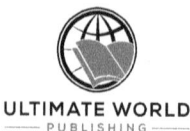

Disclaimer

This book contains true accounts of events, and all names have been changed to protect the privacy of the individuals involved. The stories within these pages are accounts of experiences of my life, and the labours and births of which I have attended and have been shared and written with permission of those whose stories are told. Some aspects of their stories have been changed to protect their identities.

The opinions expressed in this book regarding the healthcare system are solely those of the author and do not necessarily reflect the views of any organisations, institutions or individuals mentioned. The author acknowledges that opinions about the healthcare system can vary, and this work is a personal exploration and reflection.

The content and information in this book is not intended to constitute medical or health advice and is provided for general informational purposes only. Readers are encouraged to consult with relevant professionals and resources for accurate and up-to-date information on healthcare matters. The author and publisher are not responsible for any actions taken based on the information presented in this book.

Thank you for respecting the privacy of the individuals involved and understanding the subjective nature of personal opinions expressed within this work.

Content Warning

This book explores sensitive topics related to birth trauma, including instrumental delivery such as forceps and vacuum extraction, as well as postpartum haemorrhage, stillbirth and emergency medical procedures. I apologise if these subjects are triggering for you, and I encourage you to seek professional support if needed. It's important to note that these incidents are unfortunately common in the birth setting, and this book is written with the intention of addressing these realities, especially for midwives who care for women during and after a birth trauma.

Dedication

This book owes its existence to the remarkable women who have crossed my path. I've been privileged to witness their strength, endure their struggles, and share in their moments of pain and empowerment – especially the instances when they showed up with undeniable resilience. To these incredible women, thank you for allowing me to be a part of your journey as your midwife.

My inspiration to become a midwife stemmed from my sons, and I express my gratitude to both for being the wonderful individuals they are. They have not only shaped my life, they have also sparked my journey, bringing enlightenment, unconditional love and change to my life. They have supported me through all aspects of midwifery, and as a result, have become stronger men.

To my steadfast allies – my best friend Rachael Williams, my beloved grandmother, and my incredible midwife work wives, Victoria Jones and Rachael Scott – your unwavering support buoyed me through challenging times, lifting me from the depths to bask in the sunlight once more. Thank you for being present in mind, body and spirit, offering solace and keeping me secure.

Darren, my husband, your indispensable role in this journey is beyond measure. I couldn't fathom navigating this path without you. Your boundless love caught me when I stumbled, lifted me up, and set me on my feet time and again. I am grateful that you chose me.

Lastly, to the fellow midwives I've encountered on this journey – this book is a tribute to each one of you. Your wisdom is cherished, and your unwavering dedication to women's wellbeing is truly honourable. Every woman deserves a midwife, and it is your collective influence that motivated me to pen these words.

Testimonials

Wow, what a deeply raw, true and touching book is *Midwife Crisis*. All the makings of a blockbuster movie, as I journeyed through the pages, sharing the highs and lows and everything in between with Kelli and her family.

She writes so skilfully that I truly felt like I was there with her along the way – laughing, crying, grieving and celebrating every moment.

I love how Kelli shares on a confronting and challenging topic with such care, charisma, realness and power that is undoubtedly changing the paradigm, not just for birthing women and their families, but for EVERYONE involved in the birthing community.

Diane McKendrick
Those2Sisters Pty Ltd

4 time Best Selling Author
Podcaster
Retreat Facilitator
Online Course Creator
Life Coach for Business Women

Midwife Crisis

I was lucky enough to be asked to review this book prior to publishing and what an honour it was!

I was so hooked and finished reading it in 2 days, I've already told Kelli that she needs to write another book. Having worked in the medial industry and within the community, I could relate to and imagine so many of the scenarios. I was mortified but yet not surprised by some of the jaw-dropping situations that Kelli and other midwives are facing daily. This book is a great insight into how broken our maternity system is and how little the people who work in this system are cared for. This book is a great read for medical professionals, students entering the medical space, doulas and laypeople who are wanting a perspective of what it is like to work in these highly regarded professions.

Mariya Rawicki
Paramedic
Village Blossom Creator
Birth Trauma Debrief Specialist

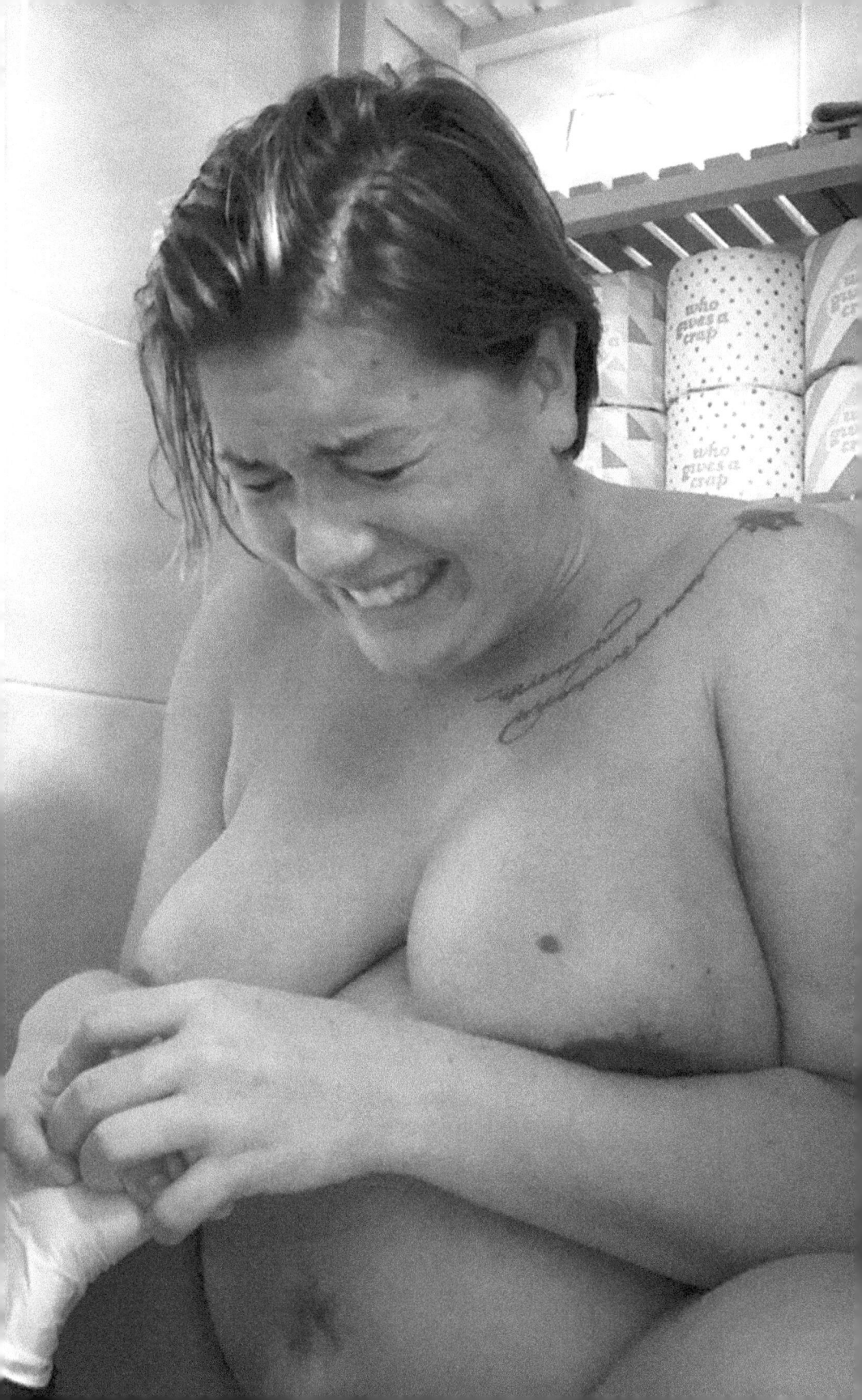

What's done is done; we cannot alter the past. It shapes your story but does not define your future. Heal your wounds and liberate yourself. Your future self deserves brighter days.

Chapter 1

I Sit and I Wait

As a midwife, I have dedicated two decades to the miracle of birth, guiding new lives into the world with unwavering hands. Yet, as I approach a crossroad of my career, I find myself haunted by questions that linger like shadows. Have I given enough to those I served? Or have I given too much, leaving so little for myself? The answers I seek elude me. They are buried deep beneath the weight of countless nights spent in sterile hospital rooms, the women I attended in labour in the middle of the night and the many bittersweet memories of lives I have touched along the way. I fell in love with midwifery – its passion, its strength, its safety. I trusted it and wanted it to support me, just as I supported the women in my care. But like any good love story, there was always a breakup and a bitter end to the romance. So, my story as a midwife is a love story of sorts.

I am a midwife. I'm not famous or an influencer. I haven't had an eating disorder, I haven't been addicted to drugs or alcohol and I had a healthy, happy childhood. I haven't made a lot of money or done anything that would be labelled a success. So, if you are anticipating sensational stories, they aren't included here. However, my journey involves its own set of challenges and 'tragedies' particularly in my career. I'm an ordinary person who in no uncertain terms, fucked it up. The meaning of 'midwife' is to be with woman, and throughout my career, that is precisely what I have done. I have been there, watching over, sitting beside, soothing and massaging. I have wiped away their tears and cleaned up their blood. I have stitched their bodies back together and I have bathed and held them when they could not. I have caught their babies with my bare hands, in pools of water in their living rooms or on their kitchen floors. I have rushed them through hospital doors, racing against time to save their babies' lives. My career has been a testament to my dedication to women, standing by them during the best and worst days of their lives. I have been through my own best and worst days, although no-one would ever have known it. This calling to be with woman is deeply ingrained in me and I did anything I needed to be *that* midwife.

My story unfolds over 20 years of my life as a midwife. It encompasses the journey of becoming a midwife, navigating through the experience and the chapters that followed. When I set out to write my story, my father brought to my attention that my great-great-great aunt was one of the first midwives in Canberra, where I was born and raised, so I guess it must run in my blood. As I write and reflect, I frequently ponder her approach to midwifery during her time, contemplating whether she grappled with similar doubts and uncertainties about her practice. Did she possess the same level of compassion for women in her care as I did? Did she advocate for them as fervently as I did?

When people learn about my profession, their reaction often involves admiration, along with comments like, 'you don't look like a midwife'. There seems to be a stereotypical image associated with midwives, perhaps involving long flowy dresses, Birkenstock sandals and the slight fragrance of essential oils. I often receive compliments about being valuable to women and people express how they perceive my job as wonderfully rewarding, assuming I must love babies, which is, of course, true. Men enjoy sharing their own version of childbirth experiences, all about how bad it was 'down there', highlighting the challenges their partners faced and the sleepless nights with the baby – and the inevitable story of how doctor so and so saved their baby's life.

The experience of birth can range from exhilarating, even described as orgasmic by some, to traumatic for many more. This trauma isn't limited to the birthing woman; it extends to the partner, other birth witnesses and even midwives. While statistics indicate that 1 in 3 women undergo traumatic birth experiences, there is a lack of corresponding data on the trauma experienced by midwives.

Midwives are often expected to just wash the trauma off, just as we do the blood on our hands after the episiotomies we've cut or the baby we had to resuscitate for over 5 minutes to ensure their first breath. We are expected to finish the shift, go home and come back the very next day as if nothing happened. Unfortunately, midwives rarely receive counselling, support or appropriate debriefing, especially after births with unexpected or tragic outcomes. Unlike other health practitioners dealing with trauma, midwives lack access to clinical supervision, a structured, professional relationship that fosters reflection, exploration of ethical issues and the development of critical thinking skills. Clinical supervision ideally is done in a protected, private space away from the work environment where support is given in the form of reflection and mentoring. The absence of clinical supervision in midwifery has a significant impact on many midwives and I believe my story would be very different today if I had been able to access support such as this.

Being a midwife is a raw and intense experience, encompassing both distressing lows and euphoric highs. In the birth room, midwives play a pivotal role in life-changing events for women and their partners. The atmosphere is charged with a cocktail of hormones, fear and vulnerability comparable to the intimacy of a sexual encounter. At times we can be observing a woman embracing her birthing goddess persona or we could be fracturing it into a million pieces under systemic pressures. It is an integral aspect of the complex reality faced by midwives.

My career as a midwife has been a tumultuous mix of heaven and hell. While it has provided for my family and sustained our accustomed lifestyle, it has also shattered me into countless pieces. Midwifery and I resemble a troubled marriage, yet I find myself returning for the passion and love of it, to face its challenges repeatedly. I am confident in my abilities as a midwife; the boxes of cards and gifts expressing gratitude over the years are a testament to that and a reminder of my good work. The women who come back for a second or third time requesting my care, also proves my worth as a midwife, and it is an honour and a privilege to care and support them once more. Moreover, it's the success of the students I've taught, who have ventured into the world of midwifery as incredible practitioners. This makes me proud and reinforces that I am proficient in my role.

For an extended period, my life was centred on my job. My unwavering dedication led me to inadvertently drift apart from numerous friends and family members. The eventual closure of my business brought about additional hardships, including having to part ways with valued employees who had become like family to me. I faced difficult decisions, such as transitioning women under my care into unfamiliar models of support or guiding them towards alternative care services due to my inability to sustain their needs any longer.

Financially, I lost a significant investment in the business, our nest egg. Being on call for countless days and nights meant missing out on numerous functions and birthdays, including those of my own sons, and many Christmas and Easter celebrations. These were all times spent with other people's families rather than my own.

My mum often tells the story that my Barbie dolls were pregnant! Cotton balls stuffed up their tight-fitting dresses, hospitals were made from cereal boxes and doctors and nurses (I obviously didn't know what a midwife was back then) helping these babies into the world. Ironically, I don't even remember owning a Ken doll then – so not sure how these 'Barbie world' pregnancies even happened.

I grew up in a very loving secure household. I had a mum and a dad, a brother 18 months older than me and a sister 4 years younger than me. I was the second eldest of 10 grandchildren to a set of grandparents that doted on us all. We were well cared for and provided for. Private schools, overseas family holidays and summers spent at a coast house that holds so many fond memories and is still in the family today. We were very close-knit and enjoyed all the good things in life.

I was part of the popular crowd at school, sporting a trendy large perm, which was considered fashionable back then. I wore stylish clothes and always had a boyfriend. I had a tight-knit group of girlfriends, and we engaged in typical teenage activities before the era of iPhones, Instagram and influencers. We hung around shopping centres, ate burgers and chips, no-one was gluten intolerant, we eyed off boys and caught buses or rode bikes everywhere. We had parties at each other's houses without parental supervision and made out with the boys we fancied until we had pash rash. We came home hiding love bites on our necks and covering up the smell of Alpine cigarettes with Impulse deodorant. Summers were spent down the south coast, suntanning in baby oil and drinking West Coast Coolers. We were carefree and had no idea where our lives were going to take us. My best friend from this time is still my best friend today and we have shared, loved and lost many things together over the years.

Like many young women, I fell in love with the popular guy at school, and we dated until we decided to get married. Strangely, I have no recollection of his proposal. It felt like a fairy tale, and looking back, it sometimes feels like it happened to someone else. At the start of our relationship, we were young and experiencing our first real love, filled with plenty of arguments and reconciliations typical of that age, seemingly innocent and naïve to where they would lead.

He was welcomed with open arms into my family. We were married in the spring of 1993, I was just 21, he was still 20. We thought we had it all, we thought we were so grown up. We had brought a house with the help of my family, and we lived together for a few months before we got married – like playing Barbies in a house that we didn't pay for. We had a big wedding. It was the first wedding of our group of friends and all our respective school friends were invited as were most of the local community. It was held at the mansion that my grandparents owned, and the ceremony was in the beautiful, lush front garden, around the fountain adorned with chubby naked cherubs. As a child, I cherished their house and often fantasised about walking down the grand spiral staircase in a wedding dress. The house featured a 25-metre swimming pool, a full-sized tennis court, and a billiards room, which we commonly called 'the pool room'.

The wedding day was truly magnificent, a bright warm spring day without a cloud in the sky. I had searched many bridal shops, even travelling interstate, looking for the perfect wedding dress. It was a grand off-white raw silk dress, that cinched me in at the waist. The hooped skirt swayed gracefully with each step I took, the sweetheart neckline and sleeves capped and adorned with miniature silk roses delicately sewn on each shoulder puff. Completing the ensemble, matching court shoes, white stockings with suspenders and the obligatory delicate 'something blue' garter. A veil of cascading tulle and lace flowed down my back, while a crown of dried flowers adorned my freshly permed auburn curls.

As I waited eagerly in the upstairs rooms surrounded by my four bridesmaids, my groom arrived in a stunning cream coloured 1950s Corvette Stingray, driving up the long-curved driveway for all the guests to see. Tall, handsome and athletically built, he embodied the epitome of an all-round good guy. It was a wedding day that fulfilled the dreams of most young girls.

A marquee had been erected on the grassed tennis court, turning it into a grand ballroom. There were thousands of fairy lights threaded through streams of silk across the roof of the marquee, tables adorned with white orchids and tealight candles, and of course there was a band and a dance floor. Our guest list had reached 200 people, and the food from the local catering company was a spread not many had seen before. The dance floor was always full and the festival of us went well into the night. It was a night to remember, and we drunkenly kissed our friends and families goodbye, well after midnight.

The fairytale didn't last long – 4 months later I left our home after realising I wasn't in love or as happy as I had thought I was. I didn't fully comprehend it back then, but just knew I couldn't continue in the façade and stay. All of sudden it was as though a light had been switched on. The marriage just wasn't the fairytale I had conjured up in my mind. This time of my life was messy, and fraught with disappointment, fear and sadness.

After many months of long negotiations we were able to navigate an amicable divorce. We split assets, sold the house and then we both just moved on. Strangely, our paths have never crossed again. It was as if that chapter of my life was just closed up and put away.

Before long, I found myself embracing life as a single woman. I hadn't been single for much of my adult life, I had fallen into a relationship and a marriage so early and so young. But I embraced being carefree and able to enjoy life again like many of my friends. I went to parties on my own, I rented an apartment and started afresh. It was exciting, scary and lonely all at once but it was something I had to do to reel back the life I had almost missed out on.

Midwife Crisis

I began work as a nanny to a family who owned and operated a number of restaurants in town. I cared for their family like it was my own and I loved the freedom of the role I played within their lives. I cooked and cleaned and managed their household. I cared for their young son and newborn daughter. Then, a few months after starting my role, their very handsome nephew came to stay. He had been living overseas and needed a place to live. The house was large enough and had plenty of room. He kept to himself, and our paths rarely crossed during my working hours. He helped his uncle with repairs that needed to be done to the house, he gardened and then eventually began to work at the restaurant at night. I stayed late at night to care for the children and when either parent came home from a shift at the restaurant I would leave. Sometimes he would come back to the house first and happily take over care. During these late nights we would often have a snack together, something he would have brought home from the kitchen. We would talk for hours, I was off the clock of course but I was so mesmerised by him. Our late night chats and snacks soon became a regular occurrence and we got to know each other and began to spend more and more time together. It felt so forbidden, but I found myself falling in love with him. At the age of 22, I still felt quite young, while he appeared much more sophisticated and mature at 27. He intrigued me with his experiences and the stories he told of living in cities like Miami, New York and Stockholm. He had travelled the world, unlike me, who had barely left the state I lived in back then. He exuded confidence and vitality, and there was something about him that drew me in. He opened my eyes to the world of love, sex and the true meaning of caring for someone. He was suave and undeniably handsome, adding to the list of attributes I loved about him.

His parents were familiar with my family, given the small community we lived in, making it a bit awkward to announce our relationship, especially so soon after leaving my first husband. Consequently, we kept our relationship quiet for a while. Eventually it occurred to me that the real reason for our secrecy was not only because of our families, it was because he was seeing two other women simultaneously! I was young, inexperienced and had only had one serious relationship before. He possessed a worldly charm and undeniable handsomeness (did I mention that already?). Not wanting to be the jealous type, I tolerated it for a while. Being the clandestine one was rather thrilling. I'm not afraid to admit that I occasionally drove past the house of his other girlfriends at different times of the day and night, checking if his car was parked in their driveways – a behaviour that might be deemed as stalking today!

We finally decided to be exclusive, after I gave him an ultimatum: it's me or them. He chose me! Thank goodness because I was bluffing. And here we are, nearly 30 years later, with two handsome and intelligent sons. We formed a tight-knit family, choosing to support each other. We have shared our lives in 18 different houses, resided in three different states of Australia and embarked on countless careers and business ventures. As the saying goes, 'when you know, you know' and I just knew we fitted together. He is my rock, my unwavering support and the firm ground beneath me when I stumble.

Our journey together has been filled with intense love, playful moments, hard work and undoubtably, instances where we've hurt each other. Through it all, we've weathered the storms, returning to each other for the good, the bad and the ugly parts of life. This is the life we chose, and he's been my biggest fan, standing by my side since the beginning. If there was a degree in supporting a midwife, he would have graduated with honours. He intimately understands labour and birth, having lived and breathed it alongside me. He serves as my sounding board, the one who grounds me, and the comforting presence that wipes away my tears when the challenges of this profession become overwhelming. He witnesses the heartache and the joy that comes with being a midwife and even after his own tiring day, he sits up to listen as I recount the details of the latest birth, moment by moment.

Midwife Crisis

As I recount these chapters of my life as a midwife, I reflect on the considerable amount of time I've spent waiting. Whether it was during births lasting over 24 hours, waiting for pregnancies to reach their culmination, waiting and holding my own breath for a newborn's first inhalation, patiently waiting and supporting uninterrupted birth or as I am now, awaiting the outcome of the most devastating event in my career. The art of waiting isn't a skill acquired in textbooks and midwives aren't explicitly taught how to navigate it. Sometimes, as a midwife, you just instinctively understand the need to wait.

Now, as I sit and await the unfolding of the remaining chapters of my midwifery career, I document these memories and share the stories of my journey as a midwife.

Being wild and wise is acceptable.

Chapter 2

Becoming Me

I hadn't decided on a career path before I had my children, but I knew deep down that I wanted to become a midwife. However, I was unsure how to pursue this ambition. Both of my children were born in private hospitals and under the care of private obstetricians. At the age of 23, I gave birth to my first son and I was 27 when I gave birth to my second son. During my first pregnancy, I was a very young woman, naïve to the system, and like many, I had private health insurance that covered pregnancy, the private hospital stays and obstetric care. At the time, I believed I was receiving the best care possible with obstetricians overseeing my pregnancy and birth. I never saw a midwife until I was in the birthing suite. I didn't see one postnatally either and I was never taught the intricate details of breastfeeding. Back then, it was uncommon to encounter lactation consultants as an external resource like it is today and the maternal health nurses were typically only visited for immunisations and baby weight. Unfortunately, many of them had poor bedside manners and would often criticise mothers, suggesting that they were starving their babies and regularly enforced formula feeding. As a result, my exposure to maternal health care was quite limited.

Midwife Crisis

The hospital where I gave birth to my first son was considered modern for its time, reputedly offering excellent food and facilities. My doctor, being the son of a well-endorsed retired obstetrician, while old-school, had a reputation for being a good practitioner. His office boasted a pinboard adorned with photos of him cradling newborns and heartfelt thank you cards – a testament to his trustworthy nature. What could possibly go wrong?

I never did a birth class. I knew nothing about labour or birth, and guessed I was just going to wing it. I was bemused with the changes in my growing belly, the movements that I felt inside of me, and I gained an excessive amount of weight. It was suspected that I had polyhydramnios, a condition where there is too much amniotic fluid around the baby. This diagnosis is accompanied with the risk of the baby not growing within normal limits, and a high likelihood of being born prematurely. It is also associated with low-birth-weight babies. The term that is commonly used for these babies is 'dropping off the perch', likening them to small birds falling from the tree branch. I was sent for an ultrasound (I'd only had one prior to this at 20 weeks) and while lying on the table was told by the sonographer – 'you had better get this baby out now or he won't survive'. Can you imagine those words being said to a 23-year-old! My obstetrician scribbled a few notes in my file, made a phone call and I was booked for an induction within the hour. As I was almost at the term of my pregnancy, he was seemingly unfazed by the diagnosis, but reiterated the words of the sonographer, that the survival rate of my baby was slim if he wasn't born soon.

I hurried home to pack a bag and inform D that we were about to welcome our baby into the world. At 38 weeks and 2 days pregnant, I was excited and scared, and I distinctly remember the first real feelings of panic beginning to rise in me. This was the time before mobile phones were accessible, so I had to wait to get home before I could announce it to my family. On our way back to the hospital, D made a quick stop at the local shops to get some food. To my surprise, he emerged from the takeaway shop with a Chiko roll, a

16

bag of hot chips, and a can of Coke. His calm demeanour amidst the anticipation of what we were about to go through, was astounding and truly remarkable.

We had spoken to our parents, letting them all know that their grandchild was on the way. D had a large extended family and the news spread like wildfire. He was fielding calls on the birth suite phone as the staff buzzed around me, drawing blood from each arm, affixing the monitor to my hugely swollen belly and preparing to rupture my waters with a long hook that looked much like a crochet needle. I was attached to a drip of oxytocin, it was turned on and up regularly by a midwife that never spoke to me, and I began contracting fiercely within a few hours. I wasn't consulted on any of this. No-one informed me of what was happening or why, and I wasn't given any explanation of what I was about to experience. I don't even remember signing a consent form. I just behaved like a good girl and did what I was told, when I was told to do it and I never realised what was happening to my body or my baby.

Once my contractions had reached the required level of intensity and frequency, I was given an epidural without being consulted. No-one asked if I wanted one or not, it was just assumed I did. The midwife who had barely said a word advised it was best to have one and that I wouldn't feel a thing. A catheter was also inserted into my bladder and I couldn't recount the number of vaginal examinations I underwent during that time, but I can certainly say that I was never asked for permission to do them. I was never told how dilated I was, nor was I told of the position my baby was in during those examinations.

Sometime after midnight, I was informed that it was time to push. I was positioned in stirrups, and suddenly my obstetrician appeared looking very official in his scrubs, gumboots and theatre hat. It struck me that I hadn't seen or heard from him since our meeting earlier that morning. A large pair of forceps blades were placed inside of me as I was instructed to push hard. Garnishing a pair of shining scissors, he cut me an episiotomy that 'may have gone a little too far' (as it was explained to me later). This is when the bleeding began, and from this point on, all I remember is a white haze descending over me.

Apparently my baby got stuck, diagnosed as a shoulder dystocia. The doctor used all sorts of manoeuvres to get him out, including attempting to pull his arm out of my body. Eventually, he was born in a blaze of glory and a whole lot of blood. The baby cried at birth and seemed perfectly healthy, albeit very small for his gestational age, and was immediately handed to D. I bled profusely from then on – D explains it like a tap had been turned on. Blood gushed from my limp body onto the floor, covering the shoes of the doctor and midwives and splattering up the walls. He says he remembers the sound of it hitting the floor. He remembers the emergency buzzers, the people in the room, who were talking urgently to each other and were yelling at me to come back. All the while D stood in the corner holding our newborn son wrapped in a regulation hospital blanket. My mum was also there, standing in the corner watching it all. D recalls all the needles that were plunged into my arms and the litres of fluid that ran through drips into me. I had passed out either due to trauma or blood loss and only awoke the following day in the same bed, in the same bloody sheets, still in the hospital gown I had changed into when I arrived. The pain I experienced when I woke up was likely the worst pain I have ever felt. My body throbbed in every possible way. It felt like I had a bowling ball between my legs and I didn't dare lift the sheets to see what lay beneath them. My belly felt flatter but wobbled like a bowl of jelly. I didn't know where my baby was. I hadn't held my baby – I didn't even know if it was a boy or a girl. My baby had never been to my breast. He had been taken to the special care nursery and fed via a tube through his nose with formula due to his low birth weight.

I mostly remember D sitting at my bedside crying, he said he didn't know if I was alive or not. He had sat there all night after they took our baby away, they had turned off the lights and left us there alone.

Becoming Me

He said he watched my chest rise and fall all night, to make sure I was still breathing. My mum, who had fallen asleep sitting upright in a chair was covered in a hospital blanket. She had been there all night, having witnessed the birth of her first grandchild and watched her daughter haemorrhage all over the birth suite floor.

I lost 2.7 litres of blood, lost consciousness and required a blood transfusion. They had pounded my uterus to contract, and I had endured a manoeuvre called a bi-manual compression to keep my uterus contracted. My placenta had been removed from my body in pieces and thrown into a bucket at the base of the bed. I had been put into a sedative-induced sleep to keep me still. I was not taken to the operating theatre; it was done in the birth room. D and my mum watched it all unfold right in front of them. They were not prepared for this. They were also not counselled on what they had seen or heard during the ordeal. They were only told I was lucky to have kept my uterus that day, that we were lucky to have a healthy baby and that the 'wonderful' doctor had saved my life.

I recovered slowly, staying a full 10 days in hospital. I only saw my baby a few times during my stay. I was too tender and weak to move out of the bed or even to stay awake. My abdomen was bruised and battered, my insides felt like they were on fire, and I was dosed up with pain killers and antibiotics. The risk of fainting was high, so I retained a catheter for 10 days, bed bathed and wasn't encouraged to get out of bed to attend to my baby.

D bathed and cared for our little boy. I didn't hold him or feed him. I lay in a hospital bed watching from afar. We called him Luis and he weighed 2.1kg at birth. He was so small and fragile, but he was a tiny little warrior that was healthy and strong. The marks from the forceps remained on his face and the outer sides of his tiny skull. His jaundiced skin loosely hung from his little bones. It wasn't the baby I had pictured in my head – all chubby and cherub like. We didn't have clothes to fit him, so my mum had gone to the toy section of a department store and bought dolls clothes for him to wear for the first few weeks. His socks came up to his hips and his nappies had to be cut to fit him to stay on. He had jet black hair, his eyes were almost too big for his tiny face and when he cried, he turned bright red, a common trait for jaundiced babies.

I was never given the chance to feed him, he had never been to my breast. He had been tube-fed formula, literally from the minute he was born then as he grew stronger, was bottle-fed during his days in the hospital nursery. Back then (28 years ago) babies didn't stay with mums overnight. They were taken to the nursery, so the new mums could get a full night's sleep, with a cup full of sedatives to ensure you did.

On the day we were finally discharged from the hospital, we were given a baby that we never actually fed or cared for overnight. I recall the words from the nurse that handed us our baby on our way out of the hospital. She reassured us that formula fed babies have just as healthy brains as breastfed babies, adding that our little one would be fat as a badger in no time. Instinctively D and I took turns most nights holding him skin to skin, neither of us sleeping. I was scared of him to be honest. He was so small, so scrawny, and he seemed so fragile. Yet, he grew into a healthy happy boy and yes, he did get fat as a badger on all that formula. I eventually did get that chubby cherub babe and he is one of the best things to have happened to me.

I don't recall much of my postpartum period: it all feels like a blur. I have no memory of receiving any kind of support from my care providers during that time, and I didn't receive any birth debriefing. I simply packed it all up as an experience and never talked to anyone about it. At that young age, I probably didn't fully grasp the impact it would have on me, both then and later in life.

Four years later, during the birth of my second son, I was induced for being postdates during the Christmas season. I had a less severe haemorrhage during the birth, I remained conscious throughout, and I fed him from the beginning. My second son was a kilogram heavier than his brother and I finally got that cherub baby I had always dreamed of. From the moment he was laid on my chest, I didn't let him go. At the time my obstetrician advised I shouldn't have any more babies, or if I did, I should opt for planned caesarean sections. Instead, I chose to become a midwife. Throughout my own traumatic birth experiences, unbeknownst to me at the time, I gained a deep understanding of the type of births I would later witness all too often as a midwife.

My style of midwifery is very different to what I received as a birthing woman. I made a conscious effort and promise to myself that when I graduated, I was going to be different, I was going to support and care. I was going to provide and ensure each woman I cared for had enough information to make choices. Choices for her, choices for her baby and choices that, maybe, would change the system. I did all of those things I set out to do and, in the end, maybe, just maybe, I cared and fought too hard and too much.

I don't often share my own birth story – it's the type of story that's difficult to recount, as it is marked by trauma. However, I felt it was important to share it here to illustrate that I have real-life experience with the same type of trauma I've witnessed countless times on the other side of the bed. I've cleaned up litres of blood from the birth suite floor. I've held women who cried in pain and screamed as they pushed against the blades of steel inside their vagina. I've witnessed women blacking out from the trauma their bodies endured during birth. I've been there too.

I graduated as part of one of the pioneering cohorts of the Bachelor of Midwifery students in Victoria. It wasn't until 6 months after graduating that any of us could register as direct entry midwives. The course was groundbreaking in Australia, but it came with its fair share of challenges. The major contention was whether we had completed sufficient practical placements during the course to qualify for registration. The greatest hurdle was persuading the

Midwife Crisis

traditional nurse/midwives that we were capable of the job. Just because we hadn't dealt with certain medical tasks like attending to elderly patients or treating severe burns didn't mean we weren't qualified. Our training focused solely on pregnancy, labour and birth and the postnatal care of a woman and her baby, emphasising our expertise in caring for women during their child birthing journey.

During my 3 years of studying, I ran a household, worked part time in a catering company and D had a full-time job at a bank. We survived with the help of my parents who had moved to Melbourne to help keep us all alive during those challenging but rewarding years. We even moved from Carlton to the bayside suburb of Hampton to be close to my parents. I travelled from Hampton to St Albans each day to attend classes, labs and practical placements. The hours were long and arduous, but I loved every minute of it. I was excited by what I witnessed every day – every woman I got to meet I attempted to make some sort of connection with. These were the days of the Bachelor of Midwifery where you had to find your own women to follow through the journey of their pregnancy, labour and birth. We had to hang around the antenatal clinics looking like a bunch of two-dollar hookers asking complete strangers to take us on their journey! It was humiliating and hard work at times. We had to follow 40 women's pregnancy and childbirth journeys during the course, and we had to attend a minimum of 30 births. It was called Continuity of Care and it was hard work but so fulfilling and I couldn't get enough of it.

I often stayed well beyond my shift to just witness a birth or to complete a procedure I needed to ensure I was competent. I was already tired as a young mum and studying and doing placements took tiredness to a whole new level. We weren't paid to do these placements either, unlike other medical or nursing students. I often recall driving home after those night shift placements where my eyes stung dry from the air conditioning and feeling high from the six cups of coffee I had consumed during the night. I often studied as I drove to and from those placement shifts with yellow post it

22

notes stuck to the dashboard. I was either studying for an anatomy exam or reciting standards of practice out loud as I drove, just to stay awake. Sometimes it was music blaring through the speakers and all the windows down, attempting to stay awake long enough to get to my driveway and into the safety of my bed.

I became obsessed with the work. It was such an adrenaline rush, being with women, seeing births, being there and getting to actually catch babies. I was consumed by it. I kept my promise to myself – I had vowed to be a different type of midwife. I read and devoured midwifery textbooks, books about birth and anytime I saw a birth on TV, I began to critique the methodology of it. I was in awe of Ina May Gaskin and the work she did back in the 1970s, dreaming the world would be a better place if everyone could birth at home and have their own midwife. I was lucky enough to have the iconic Melbourne version of a celebrity homebirth midwife, Jan Ireland, as my mentor at university. I itched to attend a birth with her. She would often come and tell stories of homebirths she had attended, but those were the days when homebirth was almost hidden and not considered mainstream care, even though it was 2001. Jan was well known in the community of midwifery and some referred to her as a rouge midwife – a name I made for myself in a few years to come, I found out later. I adored her. She was tough, took no BS and would support a woman to the end of the earth if she had to. She had an incredibly successful private practice called MAMA and she became my idol in some ways. She filled me with hopes and dreams to be like her one day. Later in my career I got to work with Jan and her team at MAMA and I took on not only one but two of her private practice models of my own. Jan, an extraordinary midwife has now retired from midwifery and handed over her iconic business. I'll be forever grateful to her and what she instilled in me.

What's in a name?
That which we call a rose
by any other name would smell
as sweet.

William Shakespeare, Romeo and Juliet

Chapter 3

Just Joey

The rose bushes that lined my grandmother's front gate were the colour of a frothy orange ice-cream soda. You would often get a waft of them as you drove in the driveway on the right summer's day. She adored them; it was the only rose she planted. The smell of these roses now, a mix of musk and sweetly baked apricots, takes me back to the last few days I spent with her. We had a bond, her and I, and if I was ever asked who I was influenced by, it would be her.

She loved clothes, shoes, shopping, fast cars and cake – her cake of choice was baked cheesecake with a good serving of whipped cream. Her house was adorned with crystal bowls full of Cadbury Roses chocolates, and she always had a few stashed in her pockets. She regularly ate chocolate for breakfast. Ironically, it was one of the last things she ever tasted on the day she passed away.

I adored her, and now my life seems to have an empty space without her. We would have heart-to-heart talks almost daily. We laughed a lot and had a few little secrets that we kept just between us. She gave the best advice about sex, love and the success of a good marriage. She and my grandfather were inseparable, and they built up a very successful business in the tyre industry. I was the eldest of her eight granddaughters and spent a lot of my childhood days with her.

My grandparents ran several retail tyre stores, with locations in the main city as well as one in a small country town, which they would visit on business trips, often taking me with them. They drove a Ford Falcon two-seater ute, branded with their business name, and little me perched in between the seats. I was a small child for my age, and I would fit snuggly standing in between them with my hands on their shoulders. Those were the days before mandated seatbelts and child safety car seats. I vaguely remember singing along with them to Elvis, Johnny Cash and Tom Jones. Once we reached the store, I would often spend time with her in the office, perched up on the manager's desk, exploring all the stationary items in the desk drawers, playing with the cash register. Sometimes, we would play hide and seek among the stacks of tyres.

My grandfather would carry me on his shoulders to the local fish and chip shop to get lunch for everyone. The tyre fitters, the office staff, my grandparents and me all sat together in the small stale lunchroom sharing the hot chips and potato cakes off the greasy butcher's paper. By the time we headed back home, I'd be covered in grease and dirt, and the scent of tyre rubber would linger on me.

In the years growing up, she was the one I went to when things got tough as a teenager and even more so as an adult. I remember the day I told her I was leaving my first husband. We were sitting in her red Mercedes Benz in a shopping mall carpark. She held my hand as I sobbed, handed me one of her many handkerchiefs and then said, 'You choose the life you want' and immediately wrote me a cheque for $10,000. She folded it into a square and said, 'Don't tell him or your mum; keep this for yourself.' This was who she was: she was generous, supportive and the happiest person you'd ever meet.

I rarely saw her without a smile on her face and a twinkle in her eye. You know how they say that a person's smile could light up a room – well her smile did just that and more. It was like a Christmas tree covered in fairy lights that sparkled brightly every day. Always sparkling and twinkling. My mum and her were like sisters, not mother and daughter. They were frequently mistaken for sisters – my mum despised it, but my grandmother loved it, and she would chuckle gleefully at the latest shop assistant who made the comment and then skipped around my mum, winking. They worked side-by-side every day in the business my grandparents had built and we all lived within walking distance of each other. I even got married in the front garden of their house. I cherished spending time with her and felt comfortable talking to her about anything. I suppose that's what I miss the most, especially during the challenges I've faced in these past few years without her.

I had the honour of being the one and only person with her when she passed away, peacefully in her own home, in her own bedroom, looking out at her Just Joeys on a warm summer morning in March 2017. She passed away at 9 am in the morning. I had been up with her all night. I hadn't showered or slept, had sent everyone else home to their respective beds for the night and I stayed by her side.

She had been without my grandfather for just over 16 months. He had also passed away from a terminal illness in the same house. She was heartbroken and she was lonely. It was obvious that she didn't want to be without him. She had suffered a stroke a few weeks before which had left her paralysed. On the day I heard she was in hospital after the stroke I had just landed back in Australia after a holiday in Hawaii to celebrate our son's 21st birthday. I immediately flew to Canberra to be with her and my family.

The first time I saw her in that hospital bed, I couldn't help but let out a loud gasp. It was a shock to see this woman, whom I had known as my grandmother, looking so different. That bright, twinkling star I adored, seemed pale and withdrawn, her mouth wide open in a contorted way that just didn't seem natural. They

29

had removed her perfect set of false teeth, leaving her with exposed gums, looking like a toothless baby.

'It's not looking good, she isn't going to survive this,' my mother said leading me out of the room in a hushed, raspy voice. Her own face red and blotchy from crying.

My grandmother was barely conscious and paralysed from her neck to her foot on her left side. She faded in and out of consciousness every few hours, often waking to ask where her husband was, and saying she wanted to go home.

'You need to help us, she wants to go home to die, she can't live like this,' my mother said looking at me with a face so serious. I was frightened, but I knew exactly what she meant. 'Again?' I asked her quietly. She nodded and walked back to the room. With a sudden heavy weight on my shoulders, I knew what I had to do and I went to find the doctor that was in charge. It was my job to get her home for palliative care.

Sixteen months prior, I was involved in helping the incredible team of the Clare Holland House care for my grandfather as he chose palliative care at home. He had been diagnosed with stage four liver cancer. He chose not to have chemotherapy and refused all facets of treatment. His wish was to die at home with his loving family surrounding him, when it was time. He was a decisive man and did things his way. There was a team of doctors and nurses at the house, coming and going throughout the days and nights, providing him with the medication to keep him 'comfortable' and sedated. I helped bathe him, dress him and I held his hand during the long nights as the cancer ravaged his body. I watched him grapple with the pain until he slipped into a coma, the medication supporting him. I sat with my grandmother, my mum, aunt and uncle in the hours as his soul left this world and all that was remaining was his body. It was exhausting and emotionally draining. But I know that my grandmother was grateful I was there. I recall the moment he passed. My mum and I had washed him, brushed what was left of his fine hair, changed his t-shirt and massaged balm into his dry hands. I recall the nurse saying it won't be long now. I whispered in his ear that he can go now and that he could go meet the angels that await him.

My grandmother had gone for a very much needed nap in her room up the hallway. My mum had gone to make cups of tea for the team of nurses that had taken their break. As he took his last breath, I didn't want to watch, so I left the room to go and get my grandmother. I recall gently stroking her thick blonde hair to wake her, her piecing blue eyes so much like my own, opened suddenly like she was waiting for this moment. They welled up with tears that didn't fall, and she gave me a faint smile. She knew it was time. She didn't say anything. I helped her up, straightened the floral cotton PJ shirt and helped her tuck it into the matching pants. She was barefoot. She went to the bathroom to fix her hair and to apply a layer of lipstick. She was always immaculate, and in this moment, she had to be at her best.

We walked down the long hallway toward the room that we had cared for him in. We walked past a few other family members who looked on, then stood up from the plush cream colour lounges as we passed them and then quietly followed us a few steps behind. I held her soft wrinkled hand tight and could faintly smell her Estee Lauder hand cream that she had put on as she exited the bathroom. I'm sure I could hear her heart beating loudly. Or was it mine?

We reached the door of the room and she turned to me and said she wanted to go by herself. I nodded and let her hand go. I heard her say so gently that he looked so handsome. She called him Mike – even though his name was Gordon. She had always called him Mike, I still to this day don't know why. I watched her place her hands on his chest, straightening his t-shirt and pulling the covers a little higher as if to keep him warm. She then lovingly cupped his face in her hands, leaned in, whispering she loved him and thanked him for a wonderful life. She said she would miss him forever. I stood in the doorway, snapping a photo of them in that moment. The last moment they ever spent together, a photo that tells such a beautiful love story without any words. My heart broke into small pieces as she turned away from him and looked at me with those piercing blue eyes and asked me to bring him back. My heart then shattered into slithers. I watched her crumble and reached out to catch her tiny frame. I held her up as long as I could while she cried the biggest tears I think I have ever seen. It was one of the hardest and longest days of my life.

That day seemed to drag on longer than any other, with various family members coming to say their goodbyes. The house that normally was filled with laughter and love and the squeals of young children was silent, all but whispers, sobs and the occasional blown nose. I remember calling D to let him know he was gone. We barely spoke as I found it so hard to even get a word out. Knowing what I had been through in those last few days, he just held the silent space for me.

It wasn't until after midnight that she agreed that the undertakers could come to take him away. She wanted us to pick out an outfit from his wardrobe for him to leave in. She finally decided on one of his favourites, a Valentino navy blue suit, a light blue shirt (which she ironed before she handed it over to the undertaker) a black belt, black socks and black lace up brogues. She said he wouldn't wear a tie so he wasn't going to be buried in one. She even handed over his signature scent, spraying it across the room as if to let him linger there for just a bit longer.

So here I was, 16 months later back in the same house with the same team of doctors and nurses supporting the choice she had made. The room overlooked the Just Joeys waving their apricot-coloured petals and I was able to catch wafts of their musky fragrance in the summer wind. I had recently changed the bed from the soiled sheets after her bowels had evacuated themselves with force. The smell

Just Joey

still lingered in the room. I had an argument with my uncle, while wearing soiled gloves – he wanted her to go back to the hospital to be cared for. I reminded him I was caring for her and so was all the other women in the house. It was an incredible moment – I felt brave, strong, powerful and in control. She had wanted this, she wanted to go the same way he did, in the same house, in their bedroom that they had shared. Not a grey, soulless hospital room surrounded by strangers and machines. My uncle's anger was palpable now, he stopped talking and he left the room silent but angry. I heard him slam a door somewhere in the house.

The days passed slowly, and she slipped deeper and deeper into unconsciousness. Just before she could no longer use her voice, it was muffled and a strain for her to talk, she asked for a Roses chocolate. The mint one. I smiled and reminded her she wouldn't be able to chew or swallow it, that she would likely choke on it – I honestly think those were her thoughts exactly. So, I unwrapped the green foil and gently placed the chocolate to her lips, her tongue ever so gently touched it and I could almost see her closed eyes roll back in ecstasy at the smell and taste of the small delicacy. This was to be her last meal. Not long after this she slipped into a peaceful forever sleep. I was the only one in the house this time. It was a bright, beautiful midsummer day. The sun shone in through the partially closed plantation shutters of her room and I watched her from the wing chair I had pulled up close to the bed. I watched her chest rise a slight amount and watched it fall, not to rise again. I didn't move when it didn't rise again, I just sat there. Relieved it was over for her. The heartache of not having him by her side every day, not to have his smell in the house anymore, not to wake up next to him every morning and not being able to say good night to him every night. She had told me a few months prior that this is what she had missed the most about him. She had held on to all his clothes, they still hung in the walk-in wardrobe, and she often took his shirts off the rack and re-ironed them just to smell the starch.

Midwife Crisis

I stayed in that room with her — just her and me for a long time. I knew I had to call my mum, call the doctor and the nurses to tell them, but I couldn't do it, not just yet. I wanted to have her to myself for a bit longer. She had given me so much, she had supported me in so many ways, held me when my world fell apart and helped me put it back together. She had listened, laughed with me and protected me. I wanted just a bit more time with her, without suffering, without pain and without anyone else around.

I had gone out to the garden a few hours before and picked just one Just Joey rose and placed it in a glass next to her bed. The fragrance was now so strong in the room, I breathed it in as deep as I could, like I was embedding them both into my soul.

I eventually got up, kissed her forehead, wished her safe travels and asked her to give him a kiss for me when she saw him. Told her I loved her and thanked her for everything she had ever done for me. I closed the double doors of her room when I left so that she could fly high and fast to the love of her life. I did the things I needed to do, made the calls, let the family gather and say goodbye. And I went to the garden and just sat with the roses.

Keep your head held up, your heels high & stylish, and elevate your standards.
You deserve the best this world has to offer.

Chapter 4

Once a Midwife Always a Midwife, No Matter How Good Her Shoes Are

Following the notifications and subsequent investigation leading to the restrictions on my practice as a homebirth midwife, I made the decision to step away from midwifery for a full year. It marked the longest hiatus I had taken since graduating. During this period, I grappled with inner turmoil, feeling adrift and disheartened with my circumstances. Uncertainty clouded my sense of identity, self-worth and purpose. Engaging in deep soul-searching, along with embracing practices like yoga and meditation and seeking solace in the company of my extended family, I embarked on a journey of self-discovery. Eventually fuelled by a shared passion for fashion and styling, my sister and I decided to pool our resources and launch a start-up venture. Together, we set our sights on opening a shoe boutique, channelling our collective enthusiasm into this new endeavour. Bonded by a deep sisterly connection and sharing a mutual love for fashion and culinary delights, my sister and I had always maintained a close relationship. While we had never collaborated professionally before, we recognised our shared maturity and commitment. Fuelled by a daring and unconventional notion, we entertained the idea of launching a business together. Despite geographical separation for a few years due to our individual pursuits, my return home marked a pivotal moment. With unwavering determination, we resolved to embark on this entrepreneurial journey side by side.

In honour of our beloved grandmother, who possessed an innate sense of style and a penchant for exquisite footwear, we decided to dedicate our business to her memory. Drawing inspiration from her impeccable taste and sartorial elegance, we channelled the small inheritance we received from her into our venture. Shoes held a special place in her heart, igniting a shared passion within us. Thus, we adopted the motto 'shoe love is true love' as the guiding principle for our store, a testament to the enduring affection and appreciation we hold for footwear and the legacy of our grandmother's influence.

What could possibly go wrong? Working on something that we both loved was such an exciting and happy time in my life. It gave me a focus other than midwifery and it reminded me that I had other skills. I recall our road trips to wholesalers in Sydney and Melbourne, filled with laughter, singing loudly to 80s songs as we travelled up and down highways in her Volvo station wagon. We dined in cute Italian trattorias, drank wine and talked into the night when we stayed in hotels sharing a king size bed, like sisters do. It was the best way to save money, to buy more shoes, of course.

Our shared passion for shoes created a daily paradise for us. With my perfectly sized foot, I had the privilege of trying on the samples at various warehouses. I would model the shoes while she made choices in terms of styles, heel heights and colours. I adored heels; she favoured flats and sneakers. It was a project we poured our hearts and souls into, and we devoted many hours of hard work – but eventually it became the very thing that tore our sisterly bond apart, and it took many years to mend.

As our business journey progressed, we encountered an unforeseen challenge: working together proved to be more tumultuous than we had anticipated. In the hectic period leading up to the official opening, tensions ran high, and disagreements seemed to overshadow any sense of harmony. The mounting pressure of our entrepreneurial endeavour began to take its toll, revealing cracks in our partnership as we found ourselves embroiled in heated arguments and constant discord. Our opening night, though appearing successful to others, was a disaster beneath the surface. We concealed our anger and frustrations from everyone else. I recognised that it wouldn't get any easier. With her strong personality, something that I always had struggled against, I (the people pleaser) found myself saying yes to everything she wanted and began to sacrifice my own ideas for the business. I soon let her call the shots, make the decisions, and take the lead. It didn't feel like it was a shared experience and as my internal frustrations grew, I lost the will to try to fight for a stake in the business. I could no longer compete with her. Despite the deep bond of sisterhood, I realised we were not compatible as business owners. I struggled with the unsettling realisation that I might never achieve equal footing in the business. The looming fear that I would perpetually occupy a subordinate role, forever overshadowed by my sister's authority, weighed heavily on my mind. The thought of never being recognised as a true co-owner filled me with a sense of inadequacy and frustration.

She has gone on to turn the business into a success. The boutique has many loyal customers, and she is well known within the industry. I do confess there are moments when I feel insanely jealous of her, but equally happy for her at the same time. Our conversations have dwindled, our relationship went astray when I walked out and I keenly miss her presence as my sister. There is an unspoken tension between us that may never find its way into words – it was another great loss in my life, of which I had little control. Despite this, I acknowledge her hard work and deserving success. I hope that one day we can revive what we once had. Family means a lot to me, and in many ways, I felt like I let her down by leaving. However, it was the first and only time I took charge of a situation that no longer met my needs. In my role as a midwife, I was never able to do this.

While my true passion remains in midwifery, I still have an insatiable love for shoes, and I take great pride in my extensive and impressive shoe collection to this day.

Following my departure from the boutique and the absence of midwifery in my life, I found myself adrift once more, devoid of a clear direction or purpose. With both of my children having left home by this stage of my life, I grappled with a profound sense of loneliness, compounded by the departure of many childhood friends who had sought opportunities in bigger cities. It took me several months to muster the courage to act. Eventually, I found a glimmer of hope when I applied for a position as a practice support midwife at a local university. To my astonishment, I was granted an interview, marking a significant turning point in my journey.

The interview day was overwhelming, and fear almost prevented me from going inside. As I navigated the long driveway to Building C, marked on the map that I had hastily printed out before leaving home, a strange feeling took hold of me. I hesitated, almost turning back, battling the urge to vomit. The stress was physical, my palms sweaty and my hands shook. My thoughts raced as I considered the potential questions about leaving private practice, returning home and the reasons for my comeback to midwifery. The fear of breaking down during the interview loomed large.

Nevertheless, I summoned the courage, donned my metaphorical big girl pants, paired with my best black heels, and walked in with the hope of avoiding any challenging academic queries. Despite my modest academic background and thoughts of imposter syndrome plaguing me, I secured the job. Perhaps it was the shoes – after all, I've been known to make a lasting impression with my footwear.

Embarking on this new chapter, I started teaching cohorts of the Bachelor of Midwifery students. It felt somewhat surreal to find myself on the other side of the educational spectrum. Reflecting on my own journey, I had been among the pioneering students who graduated from the same course it the early 2000s. It seemed like a lifetime ago that I was one of these students, with hopes and dreams of a career filled with meaningful moments, compassionate care and the profound privilege of supporting women through the transformative journey of birth.

Teaching the students was incredibly rewarding and fulfilling for me. It felt like my true calling, allowing me to share my knowledge and contribute to the development of new midwives. This experience became a source of personal growth for me as a midwife, not only providing insights into academia life, but also offering a platform for imparting the essence of being a midwife. I cherished the opportunity to meet a diverse array of women from various background and careers, all choosing to embrace midwifery. My goal was to teach them not only what they could find in books or through clinical practice, but also to reveal the genuine art of midwifery.

I'm not your average midwife and the students soon noticed this. I have a type of style that isn't what you would expect of a midwife, especially a midwife that had been in the home birthing scene. When most people think of midwives, they often picture a woman with grey flowing hair in some sort of ponytail or plait, no make-up, smells like essential oils and wears long skirts and sandals. This is not me at all. I often wear heels or cowboy boots with every outfit (unless going to a birth, it's leather Converse or a flat loafer). I sport a balayage hairstyle and I consistently wear make-up. While I often received positive comments about my attire, there were the occasional remarks that weren't intended as compliments.

My distinctive style wasn't appreciated by all, and I learnt this early on, particularly during a briefing by one of my colleagues to the newest group of students embarking on their practical placements.

Midwife Crisis

While advising the students on appropriate attire for accompanying women to antenatal clinics, it was suggested they *shouldn't* dress like me! Fifty-five pairs of eyes turned in my direction. I might have blushed slightly, straightened my cobalt blue suit jacket and shuffled my heeled feet under the chair a bit more. At the end of this briefing, as everyone began to move out of the lecture theatre, a student approached me letting me know she appreciated the way I dressed, adding compliments of my shoes and style. I expressed my gratitude and felt a restoration of my dignity, enough to confidently walk out, heels clicking with purpose and determination on the wooden floor, breezing past my colleague, attempting to show that her comments didn't affect me.

One of the students I taught in her final years of study wrote me a testimonial after becoming a registered midwife. While working at the university during this phase of my career, I received news that would profoundly impact the course of my career, my identity, and my sense of self. Following legal advice, I was instructed to gather as many testimonials as possible to strengthen my case, highlighting my skills, personality and the value of my clinical practice. Despite the significance of Jo's words in the testimonial, they carried no weight with the regulatory body overseeing and restricting my midwifery practice.

Having had the opportunity to work alongside and observe Kelli I would suggest she has the defining characteristics, of what I interpret to be a superior midwife. She is an effective communicator – the cornerstone of our interaction with people. She is autonomous – always accountable and responsible. She is in tune with normality – the physiological processes of pregnancy and birth. She is holistic, being 'with woman', truly engaging, enhancing and encouraging through forming/maintaining relationships which are meaningful within the context. And, she is woman-centred, working in partnership, providing individualised care; I would say 'axiomatic' – without question what we as midwives should be focused on. I would describe Kelli as a professional, ethical midwife upholding professional midwifery standards, using professional judgement as a reflective and critical practitioner when providing midwifery care. She is a particularly

42

aware person, including the awareness of her own moral and ethical values and beliefs, she is morally virtuous with a sound midwifery knowledge base and practical skills. She is aware of her limitations, responsibilities, and the appropriate codes, guidelines and ethical principles that guide her practice – also being aware that these have limitations. Perhaps most importantly is that she is respectful, respecting herself and others.

She was (is) not only a superior midwife; a tireless promoter of normal birth; a caring, compassionate, kind, supportive and thoughtful guide to women and their families, students, and colleagues; she also provided a backdrop of technical skills, theoretical, scholarly and literary knowledge/conversation to provide effective and safe midwifery care – contributing to the culture of the community, organisation and workplace. Moreover, Kelli reflected upon and shares professional values, attitudes, competencies and quality midwifery care to all those she encounters, thus upholding the reputation of the midwifery profession. Now, as I have become a registered midwife, I see this as a terribly important quality for a leader and mentor to possess.

Written and complied by midwife Joanne Main, March 2019.

While it is noble to offer help and compassion, it's crucial to recognise your own needs and boundaries. Take heed of those feelings that tell you something. Listen to yourself.

Chapter 5

Total Loss of Control

In my capacity as a midwife, in addition to my comprehensive knowledge of childbirth and emergency care, I provide unwavering support, making myself available whenever needed and often going beyond the standard expectations. However, this commitment has sometimes posed challenges. I have dedicated time to continuous education, undertaking additional courses to enhance my skills and accumulate valuable points towards my ongoing registration. Working as a private midwife often means operating independently, without the benefits of routine training. Being in private practice can be financially demanding, and as my grandfather used to say, 'you have to learn to earn and earn to learn'. Drawing from his success as a self-made entrepreneur, he often reiterated the importance of investing in yourself. He began his journey with a modest milk run at 19 years old, which eventually paved the way for his remarkable business achievements.

In the initial stages of my private practice, I distinctly recall feeling a sense of envy towards my midwife friends who were employed in hospitals, not because of the work they did there, but the privileges that they had provided to them. They could access training, be granted time off for it and have the costs covered. Over time as my business and financial situation improved, I managed to allocate both time and resources to undergo necessary additional training. My belief was that acquiring additional skills and knowledge would enhance the accessibility of the services I provided. I didn't just utilise resources for education and skill building; I also leveraged them for networking purposes. Operating in private practice can be isolating and attending conferences and seminars provided me with valuable opportunities to connect with other midwives and care providers. It allowed me to meet individuals whom I had only previously heard or read about, transforming what can be a lonely professional space into a vibrant network of peers and colleagues. These opportunities also equipped me with advanced skills to educate and empower women about childbirth, helping them harness their inner strength to alleviate the fear and pain associated with birth. I acquired these valuable skills from renowned practitioners, who I now proudly consider colleagues. They taught me the art of midwifery.

Teaching women to overcome the fear of childbirth can be a challenging task. It's not uncommon for women to anticipate labour as a lengthy and painful process, often with little understanding of what to expect. This lack of preparation mirrors my own experience during my births. Popularised idealisations, such as the water breaking on a bustling street followed by immediate labour and a quick, easy birth with just a few pushes, also contributes to unrealistic expectations. Births are diverse, ranging from the serene scenes of blissful new mums in birth pools with fairy lights and whale music to the chaotic medicalised scenarios we unfortunately see more often.

Even as a seasoned birth professional, I acknowledge the unpredictability of birth. The reality is that no-one, myself included, can accurately predict how it will unfold on the day. Despite meticulous preparation and planning, some births can take unexpected turns.

A particular birth remains etched in my memory, standing out as the quintessential example of everything that could go awry and

Total Loss of Control

the challenges I faced providing support when a birth becomes out of the realm of normal. Faced with the deafening ticking of the clock, she and her partner embarked on the IVF journey. Enduring numerous hormonal injections, charting ovulation cycles, and attending countless counselling sessions, she experienced countless miscarriages. It wasn't until the eve of her 41st birthday that she was blessed with a viable pregnancy.

Our paths crossed when she was assigned to my caseload in her second trimester. She would not have normally been accepted into our program due to her age, however she somehow slipped through the cracks. A force to be reckoned with, she projected a powerful aura that gave off a sense of total control of everything in her life. Tall and more accurately described as handsome than overly feminine, she possessed a striking appearance and undeniable presence. Adorned with an abundant amount of thick long unruly hair, she often used various hats and scarves to tame it and add to her boho style. Her personality was fun and vivacious, and we chatted easily in our antenatal session about her pregnancy and her impending birth plan. She was excited beyond means to be welcoming a baby. She loved her new body, her new shape and she often commented that she had never felt better, healthy and at peace with her newfound zest for life. It was wonderful to watch this aspect of her, however, this soon changed.

Our discussions focused on her desires for a peaceful, calm birth and the steps she would take to achieve this. I soon learned that she dominated decision-making in her relationship and had been fiercely independent before meeting her partner three years earlier. I sensed that they might have been more of a companion on her journey than a partner in this plan. She had an insatiable thirst for knowledge about labour and birth, seeking to absorb every piece of information I could provide. I recommended books, videos, podcasts and shared birth stories for her to read. I guided her towards birth classes and a hypnobirthing teacher I knew that could provide her with the information she sought. I engaged in weekend FaceTime calls when she requested more information and answered questions that couldn't wait till our next visit. It wasn't an uncommon approach – why wouldn't anyone want to experience spontaneous labour and birth – but it appeared to me that she hadn't planned or prepared for any possibility of the unexpected, even though this was regularly spoken about in our sessions. Placing all her proverbial eggs in one basket, executing a grand plan, where nothing would go wrong, her baby would arrive on time and she would have a natural, unmedicated birth at any cost.

Her pregnancy was categorised high risk due to her age and being an IVF pregnancy, which at the time carried a recommended induction at 38–39 weeks. As her pregnancy neared its due date, we discussed various ways to prepare her body for labour. We talked about the guidelines and recommendation of induction and the ways this would happen if she chose to go down this pathway. We talked openly about her desire to experience a spontaneous labour and that she would decline an induction prior to her due date. She had undergone monitoring and ultrasounds and received reassurance that her baby was healthy, and her placenta was functioning as it should. She acknowledged the possible risks but wanted to allow the pregnancy to continue on its own terms. She fought all her own battles on this; I was rarely involved in the discussions she had with the obstetric team who were encouraging her to go ahead with an induction.

However, at 41 weeks and 2 days pregnant having exhausted various alternative methods which some people believe could induce labour, including stretch and sweeps, essential oils, acupuncture and hypnosis, she reached a point of readiness. Despite her initial resistance, she called me requesting an induction. We had an extensive discussion about the implications for both her and the baby, discussing the associated risks. She and her partner reported that they were well informed of the risks but couldn't bear to prolong the wait any longer. It was evident that her demeanour had shifted. The confidence that she once had in her body and her ability to labour without intervention, had changed suddenly. She became fearful, and reported feeling scared that something might happen to her baby, changes I noticed had appeared following a recent obstetric clinic appointment. The mention of an increased risk of stillbirth had profoundly shaken her confidence in her ability and she now feared that her body wouldn't be capable of initiating natural labour. She started to fear her body was faulty, that she could put her baby in danger if she didn't follow the rules.

Sensing the urgency and panic that she harboured, I attempted to quell some of the fear she held but I assured her that I would make the necessary calls to facilitate her request. Frustrated, I knew securing an induction the next day could be a challenge. Fortunately, as a stroke of luck, I managed to secure a phone consultation for consent and induction for the following afternoon. She agreed with the outlined plan, consented to the induction over the phone with the doctor, therefore confirming that she had received appropriate counselling, and comprehended the potential risks and complications.

The following day, she arrived well-prepared for the journey ahead, carrying her pillow and an arsenal of birthing equipment, including her own fit ball. My colleague was to take charge of inserting the balloon that would ripen her cervix to commence the induction procedure. She would stay in the birthing suite overnight for observation and monitoring and the initial plan was for my colleague to return in the morning to initiate the induction, while I would join later in the day once labour was established. The process of an induction for a primigravida (first time mother) is to insert a balloon catheter through the cervix, fill the balloon with sterile water which over 12hrs applies pressure to the cervix to dilate it enough to then allow access through the cervix to artificially rupture the membrane of water from around the baby (i.e. breaking the water).

Everything proceeded as planned until it became evident that inserting the balloon was impossible. Her cervix remained tightly closed and she could not tolerate the insertion process, refusing pain relief. Despite attempts by two midwives and a doctor, discussions centred around an alternative method. After numerous consultations and discussions, the staff eventually reached a consensus, finding a common ground on the method they would use for induction – a pessary tape called Cervidil. However, this would require an additional 12–24 hours for the hormones to facilitate cervical ripening. It was late afternoon by the time the tape was successfully inserted. Although the insertion process is straightforward, resembling a small tampon, she was anxious, and she became distressed during the procedure, causing further delays. She was unimpressed with the situation, feeling overwhelmed by the additional people attending to her, conflicting advice, time taken to proceed with the induction and the absence of her expected midwife. Her baby was coping well and despite her dissatisfaction she settled after accepting some pain relief and the option to have sleeping pills to help her sleep that night. She was to be accommodated overnight in the ward. As I went to bed that night, a feeling of dread came over me. I couldn't shake the feeling of impending doom. It was not a sensation I was familiar with and it took all my strength to try to ignore it, but it clung to me throughout the night and into the next day.

Around 4 am that morning, I found myself unable to sleep as thoughts of her consumed me. Unable to return to sleep as dawn broke, I dressed and made my way into the hospital. My priority was to check in on her before I attended other tasks for the day. I dedicated my time to her and was supported by my team to ensure I was covered for other possible labours that might occur in the next 24 hrs.

When I arrived soon after 8 am, like a caged tiger she briskly paced the small room they had occupied overnight, back and forth in the same line. Her partner had spent the night on a fold out bed that was now jammed up against the wall. The room was cramped and stuffy, there were no windows and the only daylight came from the skylight in the hallway across from their room. With another full day remaining before the Cervidil tape could be removed and induction initiated, she was consumed with anxiety. She was edgy, jumpy and snapped at the tea lady who came in to offer her tea and toast. She had to share a bathroom with the patient next door and complained how they had used her toothpaste, she had maniacally re-folded every item in her suitcase while we talked, sitting crossed legged on the floor of the room. She spoke incessantly. She seemed to have pent up energy that she needed to expel. After checking her vitals, relieved that all was normal, I suggested that they both venture outside of the birth suite, explaining they were free to walk on the hospital grounds, even to the local shopping strip. I assured them that staying in the room was not obligatory. She would be monitored at certain times of the day, but otherwise her time was her own.

As the day progressed, she utilised her newfound freedom, frequently leaving and returning to the ward. She struck up a friendship with the front receptionist and became acquainted with the security staff. She had begun to experience mild cramps but no other signs of labour. I kept in close contact via phone and text with her through the day I assured her that I would be called if anything happened through the night. Her induction was planned to begin early the next morning.

Another night passed where I had the same feeling of dread. I couldn't pinpoint the cause or identify what was weighing on me, but the sensation sat heavily in my chest. Even now, recalling it, my heart skips a beat. I was restless and hardly slept, constantly checking my phone for possible missed calls or text messages from her or the ward staff. At one point, I found myself wandering around the house staring out the window to the eerily quiet street below. We lived on a main street, four floors above, but the usually bustling streets were subdued due to the enforced COVID curfews. Unless you were an essential worker, 8 pm marked the curfew, rendering the typically lively street profoundly silent. Not a car or person in sight, the street was so quite you could hear a pin drop. Nighttime in lockdown seemed different; the moon often appeared to be brighter, and even the stars seemed to shine with heightened brilliance throughout those long nights of the pandemic.

She slept through the night aided by sleeping pills and pain analgesia, and the Cervidil had worked, ripening and preparing her cervix. Tolerating the removal of the tape and the process of rupturing of her waters, she appeared eager to proceed. The induction commenced within the hour and by lunchtime, she was experiencing strong and regular contractions. My colleague provided me with hourly updates and the plan was for me to join around 6 pm to take over the remainder of the induction. I stayed at home 'saving hours' as we called it. Any other tasks that needed attention that day would be handled by our team members or deferred. Days like these were challenging, I was expected to relax and wait for the labour to establish. It was difficult and I never strayed far from home in case I was called in. Planning anything was out of the question, as you would likely to have to cancel it at a moment's notice.

I prepared to head to the hospital and made it by 6 pm through the peak-hour traffic to relieve my colleague. The handover was uneventful; she had barely progressed in labour, there had been some challenges adjusting the infusion to ensure that the baby wasn't distressed by the increased load of contractions. It was evident that she was frustrated with the slower than anticipated progress. The relationship I had built with her operated on a different level than my usual relaxed, easy, trusting bond with women in my care. Our connection felt distant and somehow forced.

After spending a few hours in the birth room increasing the oxytocin infusion as per protocol each hour, her contractions intensified dramatically, and she began requesting pain relief. Despite trying various methods such as a shower, using the fit ball, back rubbing, TENS machine and the gas, nothing seemed to alleviate her distress. Visibly tense, her jaw clenched, shoulders hunched and toes curled with every contraction. She became increasingly vocal, swearing, shouting and grabbing at her partner. Unfortunately, she was still in the early stages of labour at this point.

Knowing the level of intensity that the labour would get to, I summoned up the courage to suggest she consider other pain relief such as an epidural. My rationale was that it could provide her with some much-needed rest, allowing her body to relax, and the oxytocin infusion used for the induction would assist in regulating her contractions. She resisted the idea, insisting that she could cope and that an epidural was not part of her plan. However, the contractions grew quickly with intensity. Her body was becoming visibly tense, her mind obviously racing and putting her in a heightened level of anxiety, increasing her pain levels to where she couldn't tolerate any more, and she eventually asked for an epidural. Supporting her request, I swiftly left the room and booked the epidural as quickly as possible, preparing the trolley and the drugs in no time. As murphy's law predicts, the anaesthetic doctor took longer than expected to arrive – we had seemingly chosen the busiest time of the night to make our epidural request. Her pain intensified greatly during this extended wait, her screams and profanities heard down the corridors with each contraction.

Assisting an anaesthesiologist with an epidural, was always one of my greatest fears in the birthing suite. It required speed, readiness and meticulous preparation. Maintaining a sterile technique was crucial. My hands shook the moment I had to hold that small vial in my fingertips and manoeuvre it at just the right angle for the doctor to insert the needle, drawing up the powerful fentanyl drug. Thoughts would race through my mind at those moments – I had a great fear of being stabbed by the needle, or that I would disrupt the sterile field somehow causing the process to begin again, not to mention the paperwork chaos it would create.

After two attempts at inserting the epidural, a dropped fentanyl vial, which shattered tiny slithers of glass all over the floor, and a malfunctioning blood pressure cuff, the epidural was finally inserted. Once the powerful cocktail of drugs ran through the line and began to take effect, she ultimately relaxed. Her demeanour noticeably softened, and the atmosphere in the room underwent a complete transformation. My hands stopped shaking, and the sweat that had been dripping down my back ceased.

I frequently noticed a shift in my role whenever epidurals were administered during childbirth. My attention became consumed by the procedural aspects, particularly the vital observations mandated at regulated intervals. The care I provided took on a robotic quality, revolving around adherence to protocols, meticulous paperwork, and constant monitoring. In this mechanical routine, I often felt like the kind of midwife I had never aspired to be, distant from the deeply personal and holistic approach to childbirth that I had practised for so long that had initially drew me to this profession. As I did these tasks, I watched her drift off to a peaceful sleep. The room became silent, except for the soothing sound of the CTG machine, picking up her baby's rhythmic heartbeat. Freed from the grip of pain and anxiety, her body surrendered to a state of relaxation. Her partner settled in a large armchair to watch a movie, but within seconds, their eyes closed, and soft snoring filled the room. I dimmed the lights, positioned myself at the small table in the far corner of the room with a lamp and a strong cup of black coffee. It felt like I was in for a long night.

Hours passed and the induction continued with steady and textbook-like progress. The cervix is typically expected to dilate a centimetre an hour, however, this doesn't always hold true. By 10 pm she was 6 cm, by midnight, she reached 9 cm and by 2:45 am, she was fully dilated. However, the baby was in a posterior position and hadn't descended as expected. Consulting with the doctors on shift that night, it was decided to allow for what was termed 'passive descent' over the next hour, as long as the baby tolerated the oxytocin infusion, and ensuring she was not receiving more than 5 contractions in a 10-minute cycle.

Total Loss of Control

During one of the routine checks of her cervical dilation, she was counselled on the likelihood of an impending instrumental birth. This conversation also mentioned the possibility of a caesarean section if the team of obstetricians didn't feel an instrumental birth was appropriate. The consultation involved outlining potential scenarios and corresponding actions. By this point, she was tired, mentally and emotionally drained and I could sense she was losing her fight. She nodded without questioning, didn't argue or request any further explanations. She lay semi recumbent in the bed, perfectly straight, despite my attempts to help her into other positions to aid rotating the baby. She seemed distant; her sense of control gone. Barely speaking, though wide awake, something wasn't right. A strange sense came over me. The adage came to mind: you need to know normal before you know abnormal, and this was not normal now. Something had shifted in her. She was defeated. I mentioned my concerns to another staff member, the changes I saw, the way she was acting, it was dismissed as her being exhausted and tired. I regularly checked in with her, asking if she was okay, if she was comfortable, if she had any questions. She reassured me she was fine but knew that her birth plan had gone out the window.

Two more hours passed, and the baby had descended enough to attempt an instrumental birth, which of course was not in her birth plan. I took the time to explain the process to her and her partner and what it would entail. She nodded in understanding, and the doctors considered her acknowledgement as consent to proceed. The scene instantly turned clinical, resembling movie portrayals of childbirth – her lower body draped in green sterile sheets, her own clothes removed, and she was dressed in a hospital gown, her legs placed into the stirrups and the inevitable coaching from the sidelines to push began.

The first few pushes revealed that the baby wasn't coping well, displaying large decelerations in the heart rate on the monitor. A team of three doctors arrived in the room to focus on the monitor.

Midwife Crisis

She continued to push as instructed. A team of midwives and a paediatrician entered the room with a large resus cot, setting it up noisily. She looked pale and frightened. I tried to keep her focused, reminding her to breathe and rest in between, emphasising that she was close to meeting her baby. My heart raced compared to that baby's, whose heart rate never fully returned to the baseline, now hovering around 100bpm.

The first pull on the vacuum failed, a second attempt was made, however the decision was made to use a set of forceps to expedite the birth. The long hard pulls on the forceps that the small statured doctor had to exert, left me silently cursing this barbaric exercise. As the doctor coached her to push, telling her to push, to hold her breath and push harder, the other midwives began to chime in with the chant, 'Push, and again, push, hold your breath and push'. A sudden silence came over the room, the third pull, brought the baby's head to the entry of the vagina, onto the perineum. An episiotomy was quickly cut, and the baby was eventually born on the fourth and final pull of the forceps. The baby, a boy, coated in a layer of pea-green meconium, was placed on his mother's chest. He was floppy and pale, and he had not cried yet. I rubbed him gently, encouraged her to call his name, to look at him. She lay there stunned and motionless. Her partner was a pale as the baby, also stunned at what had just occurred. The cord was cut and clamped, and I alerted the paediatric doctor close by, that the baby needed support. I swiftly handed the baby to another midwife, who placed the baby on the resuscitation cot, covering the baby's nose and mouth with an oxygen mask. The team at the cot began to suction his mouth and nose, telling him to wake up, flicking the soles of his pale feet. I could hear plans being made for further resuscitation efforts. He had a heart rate and it was slowly increasing. He was suctioned again but I couldn't see how the baby was reacting as the paediatrician obstructed my view of the cot. I kept my focus on her and encouraged her partner to come close or to go to the baby, but they chose to stay at the bedside, taking and holding her hand tightly, their eyes darting between her and the baby.

Total Loss of Control

Five minutes is a long time in our world when you are waiting to hear a baby cry, an indication that it is taking its first breath of life. The baby's pale complexion soon turned a healthy pink, with the help of the expert resuscitation efforts of the paediatric team and there soon came a robust, raspy cry along with movement of his long lanky limbs. The old meconium was wiped off his skin vigorously and the paediatrician closely monitored the baby's progress, while another midwife wrapped him carefully in a blanket, placing a bright orange knitted beanie on the baby's wet head. Meanwhile she had begun to bleed heavily, suddenly the floor beneath the bed was covered with bright red blood, literally pouring from her body. The third stage drugs were administered via her IV, the placenta had been swiftly removed from her body in one almighty pull, blood shooting onto the lap of the doctor who was about to attend to the perineum. The bleeding didn't stop, the doctor seemed overwhelmed and meekly asked for help. I began massaging her uterus. A code pink was called, further drugs administered, and the room filled with medical personnel. I continued to massage her uterus, her soft moans of pain were heard and I apologised that I had to do this to her, attempting to hold her uterus in place. Suddenly, feeling her body go limp, I turned to look at her and saw her pale and unresponsive, having passed out. I diverted my gaze to the automatic monitor I had attached to her a few minutes before, her blood pressure had dropped to a dangerous level and her heart rate had begun to elevate compensating for the blood loss.

It's a surreal moment, but when faced with such situation, you often go into autopilot. It feels like an out-of-body experience, becoming rote and mechanical. Emergency drugs are drawn up, handed over for someone to administer, while others check blood pressure and place an oxygen mask on her face, someone fetches a warm blanket, and another calls a code – a code white sounds from the birth suite speakers above my head. More doctors, all senior, enter the room. Someone holds a clipboard, overseeing and noting every action in this critical moment. Another doctor takes control of the room, announcing we are moving to the operating theatre, while he moves swiftly opening the double doors of the birth room, letting in more emergency staff to help.

I haven't moved from my position where I am aggressively rubbing her uterus with my fist, almost crushing it to keep it in a tight ball. Being short, I must get up on the bed to do this effectively. The senior doctor asks about the state of the uterus, and I respond, 'boggy'. I can't get hold of it and the blood continues to flow. She remains unresponsive but breathing, her BP slowly returns to an acceptable level with the drugs we administered, but her heart rate stays elevated, and she now has a temperature according to her vital signs read out by someone else standing next to me. My thoughts briefly switch to her partner; they haven't moved at all. They now appear paler and smaller than ever as they sit in the big chair in the corner of the room, not too far from her bedside, their gaze fixed and expectant. Though they remained silent, the expression of fear was unmistakably evident on their face. Meanwhile the baby remained under the heat of the resuscitation cot, being checked and tagged by midwives who peak over their shoulders, aware that the baby won't be going to his mother anytime soon.

The once serene birth suite is now cluttered with the remnants of an emergency, with blood-soaked towels and the packaging of the emergency equipment used, littering the floor. The adrenaline in the room is palpable, with controlled and measured conversations happening simultaneously. We manage to move her out of the room on the bed and head toward the OT quickly. As we approach the door, I am left alone with her and the wardsmen, guiding the bed through the doors of the theatre. I don't look at her, but I touch her head, running my hand over her thick curly hair as I hand her over to the team who take care of her from here. I am almost relieved to leave her in the hands of the OT team. My own adrenaline is still pumping furiously through my body.

Under a general anaesthetic, her uterus is scrapped out manually, removing the remaining pieces of placenta, and she is sutured to repair a second-degree tear and a large tear at the top of her vagina. She lost over 2 litres of blood that night. Her blood pressure remained dangerously low and she was given a myriad of drugs to control the bleeding.

Returning to the birth suite I find her partner holding their newborn son. Still seated in the big chair that they had slept in a few hours before, they look up at me as I enter the room. Not saying a word they sob quietly, looking pale and weak, I quickly grab the apple juice that had been delivered the room on a meal tray some hours beforehand. I open the bottle and hand it over, encouraging them to drink. The tears streaking down their face are mixed with black mascara, leaving a trail from their heavily made-up eyes to their chin. I hand them a tissue and they quietly thank me. My body feels tired, I feel like I have done a full body workout, my abs and back hurt. A midwife from the other team pops her head in the door, and looking at the floor and the mess, she offers to help clean up. I gratefully accept her help. We work in silence. I'm too exhausted to talk, I focus on removing all the debris and blood. It becomes a priority to remove this evidence of the trauma that occurred here tonight. While cleaning I keep a close eye on the baby, still tightly held by his other parent. Attempting to make a call to family, they hang up before the call is picked up, possibly realising the early hour of the morning and their inability to speak without breaking down. They continue to stare at the baby, the perfect pink sleeping baby.

'Our baby was supposed to be a girl, one of the ultrasounds we had said it was a girl.' Their voice was shaking. I wasn't at all surprised by this statement. While it isn't common, it does happen that the gender is revealed incorrectly. We talked about the name they had chosen for their baby, and we all agree that it is gender neutral. The midwife helping me clean up, continues to haul bloodied towels into the laundry skip and begins to hum to the song that is playing softly on the speaker. The playlist had been on this whole time, but with all the chaos it was drowned out. She continues to hum along with the chorus. It's just another night in the birth suite for her.

Midwife Crisis

The ICU is an isolated unit on level 9, always quiet and eerie, evoking a sense of unease. Staffed by experienced nurses, not midwives, the unit manages patients needing specialised one on one care. She was taken straight to the ICU from the theatre by another midwife and when I arrive with her baby and partner, after cleaning and packing up the birth suite, she is awake but groggy from the anaesthetic. Gently I ask if she wants to hold her baby. She nods but doesn't speak. Placing the baby on her chest for skin to skin, I pull the hospital gown and light blue waffle blanket up over them. Observing her closely, I notice her reaction is subdued and distant, her arms lying motionless at her sides, with cannulas and lines attached. Meanwhile, her baby rests quietly and peacefully, asleep on her chest.

The tranquil atmosphere is abruptly disrupted by the entry of a nurse into the room, loudly requesting to speak with me. I step outside as she launches into a tirade of criticism, expressing her frustration that the patient was transferred to the unit with the epidural catheter still in place.

She expresses her frustration at not knowing how to handle it, insisting it should have been removed before arriving. I agree to take it out, assuring her it is not a problem and that I will handle it. I attempt to explain the circumstances, mentioning the patient was taken to theatre as a code white, but the nurse isn't interested in the details. Instead, she stares at me, nostrils flaring warning that she'll have to report the incident. With a shake of my head and a touch of sarcasm (I might have rolled my eyes before turning away) I headed back into the room. The night had dragged on, and I was too exhausted to dwell on anything beyond ensuring she was comfortable and had ample time with her baby. I was now counting the hours until I could go home. I realised I had not been to the toilet in all this time, I had not drunk a sip of water and I still had the mask on that I put on when I arrived in the birth suite at 6 pm, I had worked over 14 hrs now, which was well beyond my paid hours. It would be another 2 hours, at least, before I would be able leave. The sun would be up by the time I drove out of the hospital car park.

Meanwhile, she had broken down in tears, sobbing uncontrollably. Her partner leaning over the railed bed, telling her they were sorry, so sorry, taking their baby from her chest. Observing this poignant scene from the doorway for a moment, I prepared the equipment I needed to remove the epidural catheter from her back. The apprehension and anxiety I had experienced the night before suddenly resurfaced. It became evident that this postpartum journey would be more than challenging, requiring me to piece everything back to together again. The upcoming weeks were bound to be arduous, and I anticipated another discussion with the manager concerning the epidural catheter.

During her stay on the ward, she expressed dissatisfaction with the care I provided, sharing her grievances with several other midwives. She conveyed to the unit manager that she did not want to see me again, directly attributing the birth trauma with me. She went so far as to file an official complaint about me prior to her discharge from the hospital. Learning about this on my return from days off, my unit manager instructed me not to visit her, discontinue home care and informed me that another team would take over care. This news came as a shock, leaving me perplexed about what I might have done wrong. I hadn't performed the forceps delivery, I hadn't cut the episiotomy, or forced her to do anything that she hadn't agreed to. It was challenging for me to comprehend. It was an unprecedented situation for me. I had been preparing for the difficult postpartum visits, that would never materialise.

Realising that I had not performed well in my role was painful and difficult, especially as someone who genuinely cares about the birth journeys of families. Despite this, I had other women to care for and support, so I immersed myself in their needs.

Midwife Crisis

While she received ongoing support from the hospital's psychiatric and physiotherapy departments to help deal with her trauma, contrastingly, I wasn't provided with any support. I wasn't supported by any debriefing or counselling for the trauma I had witnessed and been directly involved in that night. I faced inquiries about my actions and perceived 'lack of care' and was reprimanded for not ensuring the removal of the epidural catheter before she went to the ICU. Ironically, I wasn't even responsible for her care after the operating theatre; another midwife took over. Yet, I was the one who took the blame.

This is where my confidence began to dwindle, and I started to question if this was the right environment for me. I consistently felt like I was walking on eggshells. I felt unsupported and exposed. I had never experienced this kind of feeling. It started with the sense I was unable to please people, not doing the right thing, and evolved into feeling blame and the disappointment that arises when you let someone down. My role as a caseload midwife usually entails a clear beginning and end to the pregnancy, birth and postpartum care. This one felt incomplete, cut short for reasons I still can't comprehend, and likely never will.

She walks with her head held high,
fire blazing in her eyes, even in the
face of fear and pain. No matter
what, she will go on, for she knows
only one way: forward.

Chapter 6

Make it Your Last

I find great pleasure in observing women, especially pregnant ones. It fascinates me to study their shapes, profiles and demeanour. I closely watch how their hips move, how their pelvis rests upon those hips and how their legs gracefully carry those bodies. The various forms of their blossoming bellies captivate my attention. I observe the expansion and relaxation of their ribs with each breath they take. It's intriguing how some women, when viewed from behind, still maintain the curve in their waist, concealing a pregnancy. In public spaces like escalators, where pregnant bellies approach slowly, I attempt to gauge how far along they might be, envisioning the baby's position – whether anterior, posterior, cephalic or breech – and the alignment of the head, flexed or deflexed. Even after all these years, I still enjoy playing this guessing game with myself.

I am intimately familiar with the sensation of a baby's movements under my own hands as I discern its position in utero. A baby lies within its mother's body, nestled deep and close to her heart. It hears her heartbeat, the rhythmic sounds of her stomach and responds to external noises like whispers, alarms and deep base music. The connection between them transcends measurement, a profound bond that awaits the baby's decisive move to meet its mother. It's a science that surpasses technological understanding.

The last birth I attended as a private practice midwife was a homebirth, a planned and very prepared homebirth during an unusually cold winter in Brisbane. I knew it would be the very last time I would attend homebirth.

It would be her first baby to be born at home after three hospital births. It started sometime during the night and a call came through on my phone. I was in a deep sleep for a change. The phone may have rung a few rings before I recognised the tone in the dark and was woken by the bright light on the bedside table. The dull shrill of the next ring bolted me awake. I quickly calculated her due date, it made her 39 weeks and 4 days, and before I slid the answer button across the screen I was out of bed and padding to the walk-in robe. In my years of experience there are some calls where you just know it's not time to get out of a warm bed and that you likely have a few more hours of sleep to get. My instincts kicked in and I knew it was pertinent for me to get up and go.

'It's time,' she said breathlessly into the phone before I even said hello. 'Okay, okay, what's happened, waters broken? Loss – clear or coloured, any blood?' I rattled off my usual questions while grabbing underwear, bra and my jeans. I grabbed the black scrub top I had begun to wear to births of recent times, only to save my own clothes from the blood splatters and baby meconium stains that often accompany my job. 'All of the above. Here comes another one, we have set up the pool.' She said as her body succumbed to the wave of a contraction. I listened and waited till it passed. They seemed short but intense.

'When did they start?' I said pulling the top over my head, phone still to my ear. I turned on the light in the bathroom beyond our walk-in robe. I hear D shuffle in bed and groan a little. He knew the drill by now. It would take me a few more minutes to brush my hair, slab a light coverage of foundation and mascara on, kiss him on the forehead and whisper, 'I'll see you later'. He moaned and called over his shoulder, 'Drive safe'. Then it's the mad rush down our long staircase, I grab my already prepped bag at the door then out into the night in my BMW. My car was adorned with my business logo, a picture of a baby and the details of our website and phone number. It was easily recognised that I was a midwife. To some.

'About 20 minutes ago. I think they are coming every 3 minutes; I get a break in between. Yep, the baby is moving and yes, I have pooed, not much blood loss but a mucous plug came out around 9 o'clock last night.' She said quickly in answer to my next few questions as I started the car, pressed the garage door to open and started to reverse out into the darkness.

'I'm on my way, I should be about 30 minutes,' I say as I punch her address into my car navigation system. It lights up and draws the blue line for me to follow, I had been to her house a few times during our antenatal visits. Only a few weeks ago, I had brought her birth equipment to her house and guided her and her husband through the setup. My second midwife, Victoria, was also present at that appointment. The house was set in an older housing estate in the outer suburbs of Brisbane. It seemed rural once you left the city lights and congested freeway behind. The house was an old brick cottage surrounded by tall gum trees and scrub, in a bushfire area. The house seemed to have an ordered measure of chaos. The usual amount of children's furniture scattered about the living rooms, toyboxes overflowing with unused toys, highchairs, baby seats and in addition a few baskets of laundry in need of folding, a half-completed jigsaw puzzle on the floor in the corner of the room and some leftover dinner bowls were on the coffee table. The busyness of their day-to-day lives was evident in the kitchen. The kitchen sink was filled with unwashed dishes and pans with last night's pasta remaining. It struck me that the curtains hanging from the kitchen windows were always drawn and had been ripped by what seemed to be cats, although I never saw a cat in the house.

Midwife Crisis

I remember stepping on a small pile of Lego that had been left at the front door the last time I entered the house and I had smashed the creation. When I returned the next week the smashed creation was still in the spot I had stepped on it.

Victoria's drive would be from the Gold Coast so I suspected she might not make it. I texted her Brit was in labour, and I was headed there now as I drove through my suburb and onto the road that led me to the outer suburbs. Victoria texted back immediately and said she was on her way too. I was happy she was going to be beside me that night, she always had my back and I really enjoyed working with her. We had a synergy between us that just worked. We are still very close today, even though we live in different cities and don't talk as often as we would like. We still have a connection and a bond that is hard to break.

As the streetlights whizzed past, the roads empty, I remember thinking – this is it, this is the last one. I had made a decision, albeit a forced decision. This was to be the last homebirth I ever would do. I had carried around a heaviness on my chest for some time and I was almost relieved that it would end. I had told all the staff that we were closing. I had those very tough talks with the clients who were due after our closure date and had offered to help them find new care providers, referring some women to other midwives, and others to hospitals for birth and postnatal care. It wasn't a pleasant experience. It felt humiliating and I experienced a sense of shame. The disappointment it caused was devastating, making it one of the toughest times of my life.

As I drove closer to Brit's house, I texted her to check in and to let her know I was not far away. She replied that things had slowed a little and I suggested she have a shower. I asked about baby movements again, and she confirmed that baby had been moving well.

I rounded the estate she lived in and made my way through the darkness towards her house. The moon was high, not full, but bright enough. Midwives lived their lives by the moons, a full moon always caused a slight level of anxiety in us, knowing that the pull of the moon often evoked a labour or two in the community.

I steered my little BMW into the overgrown driveway, branches scratching against the left side of my car. I swore, hoping it didn't scratch the logo. I'd have to check that in the morning before I went home.

I grabbed my bag, oxygen tank and birth bag from the boot of the car and headed towards the front door. Guided by the bright moonlight, I successfully dodged an upturned rusty tricycle, a milk crate and something that looked like a car battery.

The front door was unlocked and I was thankful for the lamp that was turned on near it. The door was difficult to open due a piece of ripped carpet and box of children's books that was jammed up behind it. I squeezed in between the frame and box and stepped over a laundry basket of clothes. I could hear whispers in the kitchen, Brit and her husband Dane were sitting on the kitchen chairs sipping cups of tea. I felt the coldness of the house was as I walked in. It was the middle of winter in Brisbane. There was no heating in the house other than a large fireplace, which appeared to not have been used in some time. I walked to the kitchen where Brit was attempting to eat toast smeared with a thick layer of vegemite from a blue Thomas the Tank Engine plate. I placed my things down beside the pool that had been blown up to its capacity. They had followed my instructions and placed the blue tarp on the carpet and had used an old sheet to cover the tarp, the pool was placed on top. The hose that I supplied them was carefully poised in the pool sending a slow trickle of warm water into the bottom of the pool. Bugger, I thought, they had neglected to place the pool liner in.

'You made it in good time,' Dane said to me, taking his cup to the already overflowing sink. 'The contractions have slowed a bit since the shower but just started up again.' Brit smiled at me as she went into a contraction, leaning her head onto the table and pushing her plate out of the way. Her naked belly swelled with the contraction, and I watched her ribs expand as she took slow deep breaths to work her way through it. I watched and counted the times her ribs relaxed and expanded.

I stepped closer to her placing my hand on her shoulder blades, 'That's it, let it come over you, ride the wave and let it go. One more breath, make it deep and long.' Her breath went deeper, and she followed my instruction to breathe out. Loosening her lips to breath out. I waited with her until that one passed. She slowly lifted her head from the table and her eyes shone, her cheeks pink and tinged like she had been in the sun – I'd always loved this look, those pink cheeks, in my experience told me more about a labour than any cervical examination could. It told me her body was working hard internally and that her labour was likely progressing. These are the small things that midwives like me get to see and to watch, as a woman progresses through labour. We watch and we wait.

We aren't distracted by computers or notes, we didn't need to leave the birthing space to collect equipment, or meddle with monitors. We get to see the change in her body as her baby descends, we watch her labour progress, getting closer with every contraction. I reached into my bag to grab my doppler and gel bottle, my BP cuff and stethoscope. I asked Brit if I could check on baby, she nodded and pushed back the chair, she scooted her bare bottom to the front of the chair and reclined back. She wore only a sports bra. I could see sticky clear mucous that sat in between her thighs and ran into her pubic hair. I ran my hands across her belly, found the spine of the baby which lay to the left – quite lateral I noted to myself. I then moved my hands slowly down to her pelvic brim and felt for engagement; the baby was well below the pelvic rim and was what felt like deeply engaged. I squirted the gel on the doppler and whispered it would be cold. Placing the doppler over the shoulder of the baby, a loud rhythmic heartbeat rang through the speaker of the doppler, a sound I always was grateful to hear.

Make it Your Last

I kept the doppler there for a minute or two, my hand went to her wrist to check her pulse to ensure they were different, it was a routine I followed. I knew I only had a few more minutes before the next contraction was to hit her, so I grabbed my cuff and stethoscope and quickly took her BP, everything was normal. I mentally noted all these numbers to scribble in the notes later. As the next wave came, I inquired about the colour of the loss – she pointed to a discarded pair of underwear on the floor beside her chair. The exposed pad was filed with pink mucous and streaks of blood. I nodded and smiled – this is a good sign. I picked up the underwear and removed the pad, taking it to the bin.

I looked around the room – nothing much had changed since I had last been there, except the birth pool amongst the chaos. The house remained cold, and in search for a heater, l inquired gently with Dane if there were any. He said they were in the kids' rooms, keeping them warm and asleep. I suggested that we light the fire, it was a big fireplace, and we could get the house warm if we lit it now, emphasising that it would be essential to keep Brit and the baby warm after birth. He nodded and headed out the back door to collect firewood. He came back in with a mixture of sticks, kindling and pinecones as fire starters. As he began assembling the fire, he seemed to get distracted, and the fire still wasn't alight by the time Brit had been through two more contractions.

I began to clear a path up the long hallway to the bathroom, moving aside toys and discarded clothing, so she could easily get to the toilet if needed without tripping or stepping on anything. Assuming the children were in bed, sleeping soundly as all the doors up the hallway were closed and Brit and Dane had talked in whispers, I walked to the bathroom to check for the pile of towels and extra sheets I had instructed them to prepare. They were piled on the bathroom floor, seemingly dumped out of the upturned laundry basket, which had possibly been used as a stool to reach the sink. The bathroom sink was dotted with toothpaste, toothbrushes, hair combs and clips. The mirror had been splattered with soapy water and a small set of handprints. The bath was filled with bath toys and an old kitchen pot. It was the unique chaos of the family that lived here.

I checked my phone in my pocket, noticing that Victoria had texted she was about 10 minutes away. It was 4:40 am and the sun would be rising soon, typically around 5:45 in winter. Returning to the kitchen, I retrieved my notes from my bag. Brit had stood up and was pacing the small area of lino in the kitchen. Observing her from my seat at the kitchen table, I noted her slender figure. Her blonde hair was piled into a mum bun, she had attached her TENS machine, securing it to her bra. Her full breasts swelled out of the top of the soft fabric and small beads of sweat appeared at the base of her back as she leaned over the kitchen counter for another contraction. This one seemed stronger and deeper in her pelvis. While I often ask where they feel pressure, it was evident where it was hitting her. Quietly suggesting to Dane that we put some pots on to boil in the case we ran out of hot water for the pool, I again requested him to try and get the fire started, hoping to warm up the house before the baby arrived.

I heard Victoria's Kia minivan pull into the driveway, accompanied by the sound of overgrown branches scraping down the side of her car. Victoria's vocabulary primarily consisted of profound swear words, and she likely expressed her frustration as the branches scratched her newly acquired vehicle. She was not one to hold back. Having been a midwife for the same amount of time that I had, she shared similar philosophies on midwifery, and our connection was instant from the moment we met. Despite migrating to Australia 15 years ago, she retained a hint of her English accent, occasionally showcasing an amusing linguistic quirk.

Dane finally ignited the fire, and lively flames danced around the kindling. Smoke started to fill the room, initially creating a fine haze that gradually thickened and billowed out from the chimney. I suspected that the chimney hadn't been cleaned for some time. Dane stood there attempting to fan the smoke away, and I silently

74

wished that, if the smoke alarm worked, it wouldn't go off at that very moment.

While Victoria attempted to get in through the door, I moved the obstructing basket and a few other items to clear the path. There was a plume of smoke emanating from the fireplace, the result of a pitiful fire. She gave me a look that unmistakably conveyed, 'What the heck is going on here?' I was setting up the lounge with a plastic sheet, a bed sheet and some pillows. I noticed the stains on the lounge, likely remnants of old milk ingrained into the once taupe-coloured microsuede. Victoria surveyed the scene, raising her eyebrows as she observed the smoke and state of the house.

I just smiled and gave a little giggle. 'How was your drive?' I asked.

'Drive was good, no traffic at this time of the day. Shall I go in and listen in, then?' she said as she placed her bags and coat at the door. It had been unusually cold the last few days, and she wore a heavy black cardigan, wrapping it tighter around her waist for warmth, as she turned back to look at the smoking fireplace, shaking her head as she walked through to the kitchen.

I accompanied her and briefed her on the progress of the labour. She joined Brit at the kitchen bench, where she was leaning over, ensuring Brit knew she had arrived. Placing the hose into the pool, she turned the tap on full blast, noticing the absence of the pool liner and gave a heavy sigh. I returned to the lounge to clear some more space. In the background, I could hear Victoria taking the doppler and listening in to the fetal heart rate again. The speakers echoed the sound of a thousand horses running, the beat-to-beat rhythm marked by a couple of accelerations and no decelerations. This sound always brought me a huge sense of relief.

Brit continued to contract regularly and with intensity for the next 2 hours. The contractions became longer and stronger with each wave. She had a quick nap on the lounge bed I had created by the now roaring fire, which had spread warmth throughout the rooms and created a beautiful ambient light. She soon had to stand up for a very intense contraction, during this contraction she said she had felt some pressure. Victoria was standing by her at the time rubbing her back and shoulders, she immediately dropped to her knees and looked up between Brits legs. It's an automatic reaction midwives have when we hear this, babies can just appear, almost out of nowhere. Believe me, it actually has happened. A string of pink mucous ran down Brit's inner thigh, Victoria returns to her standing and rubbing post, no baby to be seen yet.

We soon hear a patter of feet down the hallway – the youngest of the crew waddles towards Brit's legs and wraps themselves around her. Brit leans down and picks her up, resting her heavy wet nappied bottom onto her baby bump. Kisses her forehead sweetly, breathing in that sleepy, sweaty smell toddlers have. It was all the oxytocin Brit needed as she starts another contraction and quickly hands the toddler over to Dane, who was standing close by. She takes a step and a gush of clear water exits her.

'Forewaters,' Vic and I say together, moving towards Brit in unison.

'Maybe you should hop in the pool now Brit,' I say gently, holding onto her forearm to help keep her upright, as she was almost sent to the floor with the strength of this contraction. This contraction lasts longer than the previous one, she breathes through it with force. She reaches down between her legs and holds her hand there for a minute or two. The pressure must be building up now. I feel like she is holding back, just to get into the pool.

Another two little blonde headed boys appear at the doorway of the kitchen one wearing spiderman PJs that are two sizes too small for him, his belly and ankles exposed. 'Is mummy having the baby?' he asks loudly. 'Can I get in the pool too?' Dane steps forward to take his hand, still with the toddler in his arms, who still has a very full wet nappy.

'No, babe, not yet. Remember we said once the baby is here you can get in. How about we go see what's on TV?' He herds them all out to the lounge room where I had set up the bed. I hear them jumping on the lounge that I freshly made. The sun is now starting to appear, slithers of sunlight are coming through the ripped not-so-well-fitted curtains across the front windows. I wanted to open them so badly and let the sunlight in.

Instead, I held on to Brit, assisting her into the pool, her leg poised on the edge as she completed a contraction. Brit was diagnosed with a rare form of arthritis in her early teenage years, and her hands, resembling those of an elderly woman, were crinkled into a fixed position yet remained soft to hold. Despite the ongoing pain, she seldom complained, though I knew it had intensified during pregnancy. A sigh of relief escaped her as her feet touched the warm water. Lowering her labouring body into the pool, the water reached her chest. Closing her eyes, she focused on the upcoming contraction, moving into a kneeling position.

Swaying and moaning with the wave that enveloped her, she looked at me afterwards and shared, 'That was a big one, I can feel her moving and grinding on my bum.'

It was an encouraging sign. Another fetal heart check indicated everything was progressing well. Brit's sacrum was starting to bulge, a phenomenon known as the rhombus of Michaelis. I discovered this remarkable aspect of a woman's body through some very knowledgeable midwife friends, who not only imparted various midwifery techniques, but also emphasised the invaluable skill of keen observation. Learning to observe was one of the greatest gifts they shared with me.

If you place your hand vertically over the lower sacrum with your fingers pointing down towards the gluteal crease, the flat palm of your hand will be right over the rhombus of Michaelis. Shaped like a kite, it encompasses the three lower lumbar vertebrae, the sacrum, and the long alignment extending from the base of the skull of the sacrum. This area, essentially a plexus of nerves, plays a crucial role in labour.

During the second stage of labour, this wedged shaped bone area moves backwards, causing the wings of the ilea to push out and increase the diameter of the pelvis. We can observe this when a woman's hands reach upwards – usually seeking something to hold on to, her head tilts back and her back arches. The upward movement of the woman's arms serves the purpose of finding support as her pelvis becomes destabilised – a natural and integral part of active normal birth. I often witness this during labour, where a woman's arms reach above their heads to grip the back of the bed, stretch out their arms to the sides of the pool or reach up to their partners for support. It is truly an incredible sight, showcasing the opening up and transformation that occurs during the physiological second stage of labour.

Brit did this in that moment, her arms went to each side of the pool, gripping the handles that are conveniently in the correct spot and her bottom sinks deep onto her heels, she moaned in sync with the wave that took over her. Small pieces of mucous expelled along with some faeces. Victoria and I looked at each other – we knew what this meant, she had begun to push, her body was working with her baby's movements. This is what undisturbed birth looks like. I reach into the water and place the doppler on her belly to find the fetal heart rate again, it had slowed a tad from the previous ones but we knew that was also normal. The heart rate raised again once the contraction was over. Brit stayed focused and remained in the deep shell stretch she was in. Her head remained down and eyes closed. I rubbed her shoulders, massaged my fingertips into the muscles of her traps and assured her she was doing an incredible thing. 'Breath in and breath out, let your baby and your body do the work, stay with it.' Victoria leant over the pool and watched. She had picked up the notes and started to write the heart rates and the basic vitals we had taken, noting her position and the temperature of the pool.

Make it Your Last

The lounge room was abuzz with children's chatter, pencils and paper being handed out by Dad and he had prepared breakfast, rice bubbles with milk in plastic bowls. I imagined that some of that milk would be on the lounge by now.

I had fetched my mirror and turned on my phone torch to see if I could visualise any change in Brit's vagina or anus at this point. Often you get information from here, usually some anal pouting or the labia separating or the perineum bulging as the head reaches that point. I could see nothing in the mirror – I usually have to contort myself to manage this manoeuvre. I'm short and occasionally lean in a little too far, submerging myself in the water. I ask Brit if I could place my hand on her perineum to feel where it was up to. I was not at this stage intending to do an internal examination, I was fairly certain she was progressing and beginning the second stage of labour. Brit nods and again goes into the start of a contraction. As I place my hand on her perineum, I feel the bulge and the downward pressure that Brit imparts on my hand.

'Go for it Brit, listen to your body, let it happen.' I nod and wink at Victoria. It's the unspoken wink and nod between midwives, a secret form of communication that we are having a baby very soon. Brit continues to use this contraction to bear down into her body. I quickly stand and go to the door of the lounge where Dane is still holding the sodden, wet-nappied toddler in his arms – it appears she has gone back to sleep on his shoulder. He is holding a bowl of milk swollen rice bubbles in the other hand. I motioned to him that it was almost time. He moves quickly to put the little one down on the lounge and motions to the other children to come with him. The bowl of rice bubbles gets placed back on the milk-splattered table.

Victoria had positioned herself across from Brit, Brit's backside facing Victoria. She had the mirror in one hand that was deep in the water and had a slender black torch in the other. Sunlight now was desperately attempting to get through the ragged curtains. Flecks of sunlight bounced off the water, Dane went to Brit's head and buried his face into hers. He whispered he loved her and kissed her messy tangled mum bun. He held on to her gripped arthritic hands while the two other children stood behind him. They both stood silent but curious, waiting for something to happen. I used the doppler again and managed to get the heart rate from the side of Brit. Brit gave an almighty moan which turned into an obvious push, more faeces shot up to the surface of the pool.

'EWWWW, Mummy poo's in the pool, look Daddy, look, it's a poo,' shrieked one of the children. Victoria quickly grabbed the strainer (one that we never used for food) and scooped it out of the pool into a bucket she had set up. It's normal and always a good sign to us that the baby was not too far away. I reassured everyone that it was a good thing and that the baby was coming soon.

With another contraction, hitting her soon after the one before, Brit pushed again, and Victoria announced that she could now see the baby's jet-black hair. She encouraged Brit to place her hand down and feel it. Brit did and her head lifted up – her eyes shone, and she breathed a thank you to me as she went back into her focused position to continue to push her baby into this world. I stood up, grabbed my camera and started to take pictures. I took a picture of the black hair waving in the water as it emerged slowly, I watched it in the reflection of the mirror that Victoria held onto on the bottom of the pool. The top of the baby's head slowly emerges with the pressure Brit exerts, the vaginal wall expands, the labia parts and allows the head of the baby to pass, gently and easily. Victoria quietly encouraged Brit to slow down and let her body do the rest. The head was fully born into the water, the baby waits, her eyes closed. There is a pause before the next contractions. The baby stays submerged under the water, in between two worlds, and we can all see her as she slowly turns to allow her shoulders and body to be born into the water, there is no coaching, no touching. We don't tell Brit to push or hold her breath, we just watch birth happen. Brit allowed her body to take over. Her baby is born into the water, like a little fish, wiggling and almost swimming, arms and legs moving. Victoria encouraged Brit to pick up her baby, Brit drew her body up from her crouched position and reached into the water, the baby was holding up her arms to her as if to say, 'Pick me up Mummy.' Brit brought her baby to the surface and a smile so big her eyes crinkled, and she cried out loud.

'Ohh, wow, she is here, I did it, I did it.' She sat there looking at her baby for what seemed like an eternity, the baby opened her eyes, coughed a little and let out a little cry, she was breathing and I reached down to check her cord was pulsing. It was beating perfectly and the baby had snuggled herself into Brit's chest.

In my experience of women birthing in water, the baby often appears blue when they are first born, which is a normal physiological response to having been born under water. The Apgar score we use to assess their respiration, tone and colour within the first minutes of birth, tells us if we would need to act to supply oxygen, but with the stimulation from their mother touching and rubbing them, they turn pink fairly quickly. We helped Brit into a more comfortable position leaning back against the pool's seat and covered her and the baby with towels to keep them warm. The room was now warm from the fireplace and I had also turned on the oven to help heat the space up (another little hack midwives do to keep houses warm). During my assessment of the baby, including feeling the cord for pulsations, the pink, alert baby lifted her head and looked her mother in the eyes, assessing she was safe and sound on the outside.

'I almost didn't think I could do that,' Brit said as she kissed her newborn baby on her slick wet head. 'It's a girl' none of us had actually looked but we did check and announced it was a girl.

Dane hadn't said a word through this, I think he was in awe of what he had witnessed. The kids were also unusually quiet, but we did hear a whimper from the other room from the toddler that had been left in her wet nappy on the lounge. He quickly got up to get her. She reached out for her mummy when she was carried into the room and he whipped off that soaked nappy and her PJs and placed her in the pool beside Brit and her newborn sister.

'Me too Daddy,' said the other one, with his pants down already, arms up, asking to be placed in the pool.

I settled back on my heels, inhaling a slow, deep breath that helped calm my racing heart. A tightness in my chest, often accompanying tears, emerged, but I suppressed the emotions, offering a smile. I observed a family meeting their new sister, the sun casting a warm glow across the pool, while the fire crackled and spat embers on the brick hearth. It was the last homebirth I would ever attend. I was grateful beyond measure that Victoria had been by my side that day. She was my anchor of calm.

The weight of the moment didn't fully hit me until I pulled into my garage later that day. Sitting in my car, I pressed the button to lower the garage door, enveloping myself in darkness. I turned off the car and allowed myself to cry – the kind of deep, ugly crying that lasted a solid 15 minutes. I shed tears for the end, for what I had achieved, and for the unknown chapter awaiting me. As I wiped my face with my sleeve and a previously used tissue from the console, I noticed the lingering smell of campfire on my clothes. My phone pinged – it was Victoria. She had gotten home, shared a similar experience with the campfire scent and mentioned discarding her cardigan officially by burning it. Her familiarity and humour changed my mood. Gathering up my belongings, I walked inside, greeted my family with a big smile and embraced the transition ahead of me.

Dreams become reality, not through chance, but through relentless effort, unwavering determination, and the hard work that bridges the gap between aspirations and achievements.

Chapter 7

Dreams Do Come True

My dream finally came true. You know those people who use visualisation to manifest what they want? With the vision boards, the meditation and mantras? Well, I'm not one of those people. I just do things – I think about it and I get it done. I had a thought one day to set up a clinic where I could work, bringing all the practitioners that I had already began to refer my clients to, all in one place. A place that was homely, easy to access, with rooms for each practitioner to work from, creating a space and a place for women to meet other women and to ensure their care was all in one spot. A one-stop-shop so to speak. I made a call to my trusty friend and advocate for all things midwifery Jan Ireland. Jan operated a service in Melbourne called MAMA – Midwives and Mothers Australia. I was in awe of what she had created. It was exactly what I wanted to do. I had to find a way to replicate it. We discussed my plans and she invited me to meet with her and her business partner to discuss it further.

Two days later I was on a flight to Melbourne. A few weeks later we were setting up MAMA Brisbane. Jan agreed for me to use the name and business model. I already had the practitioners on stand-by and spent the next 2 weeks finding the perfect place to house my MAMA. The vision I had was homely, plenty of room and close to the major aspects of Brisbane city.

I committed a significant portion of our savings to the business, taking a calculated risk based on strong belief and the need for such a facility. Brisbane had not seen a place of this calibre before. We finally found the perfect place to secure as our MAMA Centre, as we so fondly called it.

With the assistance of Ikea, D, and his adept use of a drill set, we employed creative building techniques to actualise the space I had envisioned. Converting an old Queenslander-style house into an office, we strategically organised its five rooms. Downstairs, two rooms were tailored for the chiropractor and massage therapist, with an expansive area designated for yoga classes. A welcoming reception area was crafted, while upstairs, three rooms were allocated for the midwives, naturopath and acupuncturist. Our future plan involved accommodating a GP specialist or lactation consultant once the business gained traction. The facility boasted a kitchen and two bathrooms. The midwives' rooms were tastefully adorned with calming, teal-coloured lounges, complemented by a white work desk, chairs and baby weighing stations.

I assembled my dream team to help manage and execute this extraordinary place. Initially I connected with a midwife who eventually became my business partner, although regrettably, our partnership didn't end well. During my years as a midwife, I had been referring my clients to a variety of allied health professionals. I gathered them all together in my own living room one day and proposed the idea of joining MAMA Brisbane. To my delight, they all eagerly accepted the opportunity. It was a perfect synergy and plan. We collaborated to create a business model that suited everyone, and within a few weeks we were all working from the MAMA Centre.

Dreams Do Come True

We stocked the drawers with dopplers, pinards, tape measures, pregnancy wheels and the essential pathology equipment for bloodwork. Pastel artwork and midwifery and birthing books adorned the space. I painstakingly curated pictures of women who had birthed with me over the years and placed these in small black picture frames that hung at various angles along the walls of the staircase. I even hung an oversized paper chandelier from the 17-foot ceiling above the staircase.

The unusually spacious lounge at the top of the stairs was divided by flowing white curtains, with plush grey sofas for pregnant women to relax in. Matching wing chairs, pastel-coloured rugs on the floor and scattered white coffee tables completed the cosy ambience. The kitchen adopted a self-serve concept, equipped with a pod coffee machine, a variety of herbal teas and a perpetually overflowing fruit bowl and biscuit jar. This space hosted weekly mothers' groups and served as the venue for our hypnobirthing and active birth classes.

Introducing new clients to this space always brought joy, as they consistently expressed appreciation for the welcoming atmosphere, often commenting on how much it felt like 'home'. My office served as my sanctuary, a space I cherished for its solitude. Whether during early mornings, late nights or occasionally in the middle of the night after attending a birth too far from home, I sought refuge here in the clinic to unwind and simply be.

Having initiated my practice from home a couple of years prior, transitioning to the clinic was seamless, as I wasn't starting from scratch. Introducing my clients to the clinic space and the accessibility to other practitioners brought me immense joy. Families started coming in, phones rang, bookings increased, and we settled into a daily rhythm. Our plan was to ensure that women had at least three points of contact in the clinic. They could consult with their midwife, see the chiropractor, have a massage, visit the naturopath or participate in a yoga class. This structured program allowed us to cover expenses and generate a profit easily. In addition to these core services, we offered various extras such as placenta encapsulation, sleep and settling techniques for young babies, breastfeeding support, tongue tie assessment and revisions. Our shelves were stocked with a variety of pregnancy and birth books, essential oils and lactation cookies, which regularly sold out. The clinic became a go-to destination for anything related to pregnancy and postnatal care. It embodied the essence of midwifery dreams, truly standing as a place that was with women every step of the way.

Our homebirth inquiry rates saw a significant increase and with the establishment of the clinic we introduced the option for clients to receive midwife support in a hospital setting. I was granted eligibility as a midwife to provide care in hospitals, a ground-breaking development in Queensland, making it the first state to allow private midwives to attend their clients in hospital. This became a major attraction for the business.

Our homebirth to hospital birth ratio settled at 80/20, and we maintained a low transfer rate. Offering Medicare rebates and becoming a preferred private health insurance provider for additional healthcare services, further solidified our position in the market of woman-centred care providers. It truly felt like a dream had come true for me.

The clinic became a safe place for women to come to receive nurturing and non-clinical care. I also used it as my safe place, as there were times when I didn't want to head straight home, preferring to avoid conversations about the births I had witnessed. I yearned for a space where no-one would touch or talk to me. On one particularly exhausting night after a lengthy day and night of labour and birth, I curled up on the lounge in my office – a place of silence and safety. I loved my family and knew I should go home, but there were times when I just needed to switch off from being everything. Drifting off to sleep for a few hours, I awoke to the sun peeping through the slatted blinds and the warmth of the day creeping in. I texted D to let him know I was on my way home, never mentioning I had spent the night at the clinic.

About a year into operating the clinic, we experienced a break-in one night, with intruders likely seeking drugs, breaking through one of the downstairs wooden doors. They ransacked the place, taking only a few handfuls of breastfeeding syringes. Upon receiving the call from the security company, D and I rushed to the clinic to find the door off its hinges, leaving the place vulnerable and unsecured. Bravely, we decided to stay the night, fearing the possibility of the burglars returning. Neither of us slept well, as we anxiously jumped at every noise and every creak the old house made, nervously needing to protect our livelihood and assets.

I found myself navigating a whirlwind of adrenaline and exhaustion as the business took off, as I juggled the clinic, overseeing staff, attracting new clients and attending births around the clock. It became clear I needed a practice manager to alleviate the load. I had recently connected with a new client who was in the early stages of her pregnancy and planning a homebirth with us. She had all the attributes of the perfect practice manager. We connected on business ideas and I saw an opportunity to offer her a part-time role until her baby was born. She accepted and with her handling many aspects of the day-to-day clinic management I began to breathe a little easier.

The second year brought some challenges as we expanded with a new clinic on the Sunshine Coast, demanding considerable attention and care. Simultaneously, the relationship with my business/midwife partner began to unravel. Disagreements surfaced regarding fundamental aspects of the business. We attempted to salvage the partnership, but it proved unsuccessful, leading to a contentious separation. I went on to run the business on my own, eventually engaging more midwives and forming a tight knit team of support around me. Amidst this turmoil, the late stages of 2016 presented a situation that deeply shook my world, soul and the very core of the business.

Giving birth is both beautiful
and brutal, an experience that
cracks you open and takes you
to places you never knew existed,
transforming you into a mother
with a depth of love and strength
you never imagined possible,
without an instruction manual.

Chapter 8

Jumping Puddles

Being on call is not just a facet of private practice; it also became a defining aspect of my life during my time in a group practice within a hospital. It is arduous, relentless, and ironically, it is what I loved about being a midwife. This set-up freed me from the constraints of shift work, the routine of showing up to the same shift, with the same team, and attending the same inductions day after day. Being on call offers a level of freedom, allowing me to change my schedule daily. It provided flexibility to have days at home, spend time with D and the boys, attend school sports days or concerts, and enjoy lunches or dinners with friends. However, each invitation or plan I made came with the preface, 'I'm on call, so I may have to leave halfway through or not make it at all.' D and I often took two cars to events so that I could leave if needed. I've answered calls in the middle of dinners, weddings and even Christmas days. It's a profession that doesn't take holidays into account.

I remember one Christmas morning during my private practice days when we had planned for some friends to come over for breakfast. We had laid out some beautiful food and a couple of bottles of champagne to celebrate the festive season. I (of course) was on call, so not drinking. Our friends wanted to show us their Christmas present that they had gotten for each other. It was a surprise, so we were excited to see what it could be. Perhaps a new car, or a diamond ring? They showed up laden with brightly wrapped gifts and food, and as usual, both were immaculately dressed.

Jayne had a tight-fitting black mini dress with an elaborate gold zipper that ran the length of the dress. She paired it with gold stilettos that wrapped up her ankles. She never went anywhere without a good pair of heels. Joe was dressed in a blue paisley three-piece suit and shiny bright blue shoes. This was his usual dress sense at any time of the day. They were quite an eccentric couple that we dearly loved and had known for a long time.

I hadn't received a call overnight, so I felt secure enough to proceed with the plan of having breakfast and later, lunch with other friends. When our friends arrived, we clinked champagne flutes and began to eat. About 30 minutes into their visit, my phone rang – it was one of my Sunshine Coast clients. She informed me that she had experienced a few contractions in the night, which had settled but now were starting again. She wanted to keep me informed, considering the drive from Brisbane. She had plans for a brunch with family and was hoping to go home and have a nap at some stage. Despite her hopes, I had an inkling that she wouldn't be making that nap. I asked her to call me back in an hour to update me. I informed my friends once I hung up that I would likely be leaving soon – a familiar mix of disappointment, empathy and excitement crossed their faces, knowing that I would be leaving them to attend a birth. The call came before the hour had passed, that her contractions had indeed ramped up to 5-minute intervals.

As I prepared to depart, they reminded me that they hadn't shown us their surprise Christmas present. I was distracted, getting things into my car, so I wasn't paying too much attention. Jayne grabbed me by the hand and pulled me into the kitchen. She stood squarely in front of me, unzipped the gold zipper to her waist, revealing her newly augmented breasts. I had to blink a few times. They were round and perky, shiny and tight, with pink nipples standing up, looking straight at me. She was once an A cup, if that, but these were verging on double DDs.

'Ta daa,' she said with her signature giggle. 'Do you like them?'

So, this was the surprise. D walked in, stopped mid-step and had a perplexed look on his face. He was holding two glasses of champagne, casually handed one to Jayne, nodding with gratitude.

'I like them. These were the Christmas present?' He enquired, cocking his head to one side, inspecting her chest. Jayne happily nodded and the newly augmented boobs bobbed a little. They were still so fresh, so there was not too much movement.

Joe raised his glass and chimed in. 'Yeah, they are great, aren't they? We knew you would appreciate a good set, Kel. Merry Christmas everyone.' Jayne finally zipped up her dress, took a sip from her champagne flute, gave me a wink, kissed me on the cheek and wished me a very Merry Christmas. I was still a bit dazed and went about getting ready to head off. My phone rang again as I made my way out to the car.

I waved goodbye to everyone and winked at D, hoping he would enjoy his day. I had encountered many breasts before, having held them, massaged them, soothed the red lumps out of them and even tweaked a few nipples in my time. However, this was a sight to behold in my own kitchen on Christmas Day. Once in the car and on my way, I continued to smile and shake my head. I love my friends and love that they trust me enough to show me their new beaming assets.

Cruising down the highway towards the coast, I constantly received text message updates on how she was doing. Contractions had ramped up, she was still managing to sit at the Christmas table with the family, occasionally wincing and discreetly breathing through the more biting ones. As I was exiting the highway towards the Sunshine Coast University building, the phone rang. Thank goodness for speaker phones.

'My waters just broke at the table. I'm sitting in a puddle right now and my mother-in-law is getting towels to mop it up. Do you think we should leave for the hospital now?' she speaks in a fast high-pitched tone.

'Sounds like a good plan. I'll meet you there, I've just passed the Uni, it will take me about 20 more minutes. Call the hospital and let them know you are coming and I'm on my way.'

'Great, we are all pack…ed!' her voice hit a high note as a contraction came over her. I could hear a commotion in the background like chairs being pushed back on the floorboards, lots of excited chatter and there were a few children squealing in the foreground.

'Okay please call me on the way if anything changes.' I pressed the end key and pushed the BMW a little bit harder. Christmas Day on the coast was usually quiet so there weren't too many other cars on the road. The journey typically took well over an hour, but that day I trimmed it down to 50 minutes. With adrenaline coursing through my veins, the drive was smooth and effortless, the roads clear and devoid of traffic along the tranquil streets. Upon reaching the hospital, I parked in the visitor's lot and made my way inside. By now, I had become familiar to the reception staff, wishing them all a Merry Christmas. I was waved through to the birth suite. The walls and ceiling were adorned with Christmas decorations, and a large tree lit up with brightly coloured lights, reminded me of the significance of the day. The receptionist informed me that my client had already arrived and was in active labour, gesturing towards room 2. Despite lacking visiting rights at this private hospital, I was welcomed as a support person.

Jumping Puddles

The maternity unit embraced water births, a pioneering concept on the coast at the time, and she had already immersed herself in the large round pool at the centre of the room. Each woman was assigned a private obstetrician and care was shared between the hospital and private midwives, reflecting a progressive and woman-centred approach to maternity care. I always felt embraced here, part of the team, and my skills valued.

Her labour had progressed rapidly, she was already pushing when I entered the room. Quietly I crouched beside the attending midwife, gently signalling my presence. She made room for me at the edge of the birth pool and handed me the doppler to monitor the fetal heart rate. Leaning in, I whispered reassuringly as I checked on the baby, that she was doing so well. With a powerful push, the occiput of the baby's head began to emerge, jet-black hair swaying in the water. She continued with her pushing efforts and more of the head was birthed into the water. I watched its cheeks and then the chin emerge. I was able to see this incredible moment in the mirror the other midwife was holding. My eyes locked with hers as I offered words of encouragement, assuring her that she was doing wonderfully and that her baby was almost here. As the baby smoothly slipped into the warm water, I encouraged her to reach down to bring her newborn to her chest. In an instant, she brought her baby to the surface and cradled him to her chest. He took his first breath as she kissed his wet head. The midwife beside me hummed a Christmas carol and soon we all joined in, celebrating the birth of a Christmas Day baby. Though I missed spending the day with my own family, witnessing the joy of a new family filled with me warmth and pride. I didn't return home until later that night, knowing that I could celebrate Christmas another day.

It's commonly known that second labours tend to be faster, a fact I've found to be true in my experience. Second labours are often shorter than the first, with the increased likelihood of spontaneity and minimal intervention. Many second time parents are surprised by the intensity and speed of second labours, having expectations

Midwife Crisis

similar to that of their first. Stories of second births occurring unexpectedly, in elevators, at the doors of birthing suites, in cars, at home in bathrooms or showers and even on the side of the road are relatively common.

One summer day a client contacted me, having experienced a long first labour with her previous child, which had extended well beyond her due date. She anticipated her labour to be at least 2 weeks away, unaware that her body had already begun preparing. She had a deep sleep that night and had awoken feeling fresh with no signs of labour. She had begun, unbeknown to her, to secrete that lovely hormone of oxytocin that causes the feeling of euphoria in women just before labour begins. They were celebrating her grandmother's 80th birthday that day and she had volunteered to hold the party at her home. She had cooked up a feast and was looking forward to seeing family and friends, including some relatives who were coming from out of town.

She floated around the house early that morning, cleaning and setting the table. She had been out in the garden before the rest of the family had woken and picked fresh flowers, placing them in vases down the centre of the table.

As the morning went on, she felt some mild tightness, associating it with the movements of the baby. She would rub her belly occasionally and fondly refer to her little one as 'jellybean'. As the house began to fill with family and friends around midday, the children happily playing and running around, she felt the first pangs of contractions. Heading to the toilet she noticed the mucous plug had dislodged itself, leaving a small stain of pink on her underwear. It was too late to call off the party now, she would just have to get through it. Surely her labour wouldn't happen today, she kept telling herself.

Sending me a text from the bathroom, she told me of the pink staining and the mild tightenings she was having. I let her know I was available that day and when she needed me to ensure she gave me notice as I would be travelling from Brisbane to the coast. We agreed that she should update me with any contractions that became regular. I didn't hear back from her until later in the day.

Her party guests arrived and enjoyed the feast she had laid out on the table. The children played in the sunshine with bubbles and the use of the new trampoline. As she sat at the table enjoying dessert, she felt a sudden urge to go to the toilet. Excusing herself, she rushed to the bathroom and felt a gush of warm fluid, signalling her waters had broken. Unsure of what to do next, she called me, whispering her situation over the phone. We agreed that I would travel to the coast, and she would update me on her contractions and progress.

Going back to her seat and sitting next to her aunt, she felt another gush of water into the pad she was wearing, it didn't hold it, spilling out and over it onto the cushion of the chair. Sitting in the wetness, she focused on the intense wave that ripped through her, beginning in her back and moving its way to the front of her pelvis. She was in denial, there is no way this could be happening this fast, her last labour had taken 28 hours. She eventually got out of the seat with help from her very concerned husband, paddled her way to the bathroom to change her underwear and clothes. Three more intense contractions hit her, causing her to hold onto the bathroom bench for support. Texting me in between the contractions, she alerted me that they had come on strong and that she would head to hospital. Texting her husband from the bathroom, she asked him to get her bags into the car. Appearing in the doorway, he looked concerned.

'Are we having the baby now, right now?' he asked. 'Yes, let's go,' is all she could get out. Moving slowly out of the bathroom and towards the kitchen (she didn't want to face the guests) she took the route through the laundry to the garage. As she navigated the stairs to the garage, he rummaged up the bags, told the guests they would be back and scooted out the front door, meeting her in the cool dark garage at their car. She told him they needed to hurry.

Midwife Crisis

Backing out carefully so they did not hit any of the guests' cars that lined the driveway, they turned onto the main road that took them to the highway. The hospital was approximately 30 minutes from their rural hinterland home. Rolling green hills and wide-open spaces were on either side of the road that led to the highway. Her contractions had intensified once more and she began to feel a pressure she had not experienced before. She let out a moan when the next contraction hit her, deep in her pelvis radiating into her backside. She had not been able to put on new underwear so was naked under her sundress.

Telling him that she didn't think she would make it, she asked him to stop the car. Confused by what she meant, he began questioning her, obviously not understanding what she meant.

'The baby is coming,' she said, holding her hands between her legs, feeling so much pressure it was hard to ignore now. She felt her body bearing down into the depths of the car seat. The seatbelt was cutting into her hips. Releasing it, she moved to a more upright position.

He slowed the car, indicating that he was pulling off the road. As soon as the car came to a stop, she stepped out, as another bearing down contraction took over her body. She walked to the grass, squatting instinctively. As he came around to the other side of the car, he saw someone on a ride-on mower not too far in the distance on the property. Waving at the man, he began to run towards him. They ran back to her together. The man introduced himself as a vet, commenting that he had helped deliver calves but never a baby. She squatted between the two of them and began to push her baby out into the world in that stunning green paddock. Her baby was born into the hands of the vet as her husband looked on in wonder and in complete shock of what was happening. Sitting on the grass holding her newborn son who was pink and crying, she was covered in a towel that had been found it the back of the car, and the baby loosely wrapped in the flannel shirt the vet had been wearing. The three of them could hardly believe what had just occurred. Leaning in, her husband asked if he should call the midwife. She nodded and said I'd likely be on my way and at the hospital by now. As I was approaching the gates of the hospital, the phone rings again, displaying her name on the screen. This time, Luke is on the line, his voice crackling as he speaks rapidly. 'Kel, we didn't make it. We're on the side of the road, the baby is born. A local vet came and helped us. She is okay. We will head into the hospital now. Or wait, should we call an ambulance?' I chuckled at his excitement and nervousness. I could just imagine the adrenaline running through him at that moment.

'How wonderful! Yes, call an ambulance, stay where you are, they will come and get you. Well done. Put me on speaker.' I spoke to them both and congratulated the vet for his efforts. We assessed the condition of the baby and how to keep him warm and out of the sun. I advised them I was already at the hospital and would await their arrival. I was so proud of her, of them both. It was a remarkable effort, and I am sure the experience was quite intimidating for them. Her previous birth had been a prolonged labour where she had been induced for post-dates, ending in a vacuum extraction and a third-degree tear.

The buzz of excitement was soon dulled by some snide remarks made from the ward midwives, suggesting that they should have left home earlier to avoid the predicament they had found themselves in. It was fortunate that they had seen the vet and he assisted them. He kept them calm, helped her into a squat position and played a crucial role in catching their baby. She relied on her instincts, tapping into the connection between her body and her baby, guiding her to a safe birthing space.

The on-call work of a midwife can be gruelling, but in turn very rewarding. I recall a home birth where I stayed with the couple for over 34 hours straight. Managing short naps and switching out shifts with my midwife partner, it was an intense experience that I couldn't turn off from. Dealing with a mispositioned baby, it required all our expertise to assist in repositioning, allowing us to avoid transfer to the hospital and unnecessary interventions. She was incredibly resilient and determined, pushing herself to a remarkable extent that astonished even me. Eventually she birthed her baby on the lounge room floor, following her own timeline and terms. It was the unwavering determination of women like her that fuelled my commitment to this work.

Birth doesn't adhere to a schedule; it can happen at any time of the day or night, including weekends, and public and religious holidays. However, a weekday midday birth is a rarity. I once attended one of these rare occasions, a fast and furious first labour where the baby needed a few minutes of extra oxygen for a smooth transition into the world. Both the second midwife and I had parked our cars across the road from the house. After the birth we packed up and I stayed on to help settle them into bed for the afternoon. It was 4 pm when I happened to glance out the front window and saw my car being lifted onto a tow truck. I had parked in a clearway. Panic set in as I raced outside, waving and yelling at the tow truck driver, who looked remarkably like Mike Tyson. I begged him not to tow my car, explaining that I was a midwife at the house where we had just welcomed a new baby. It took some convincing, but I managed to retrieve my car after paying him a handsome $500 fee. It certainly was a close call that day, on multiple fronts.

Being a midwife on call doesn't come with any special privileges either, especially not speeding privileges. Given the nature of my work, which involves a considerable amount of driving, I opt for cars that are fast, often turbo-boosted, reliable and capable of carrying a substantial amount of equipment like birthing pools, oxygen tanks and birthing bags filled with essential supplies. At one point, I even had my logo and business name 'MAMA Midwife' splashed across my car in bright green. Many times, I received a thumbs up or gestures from people at traffic lights or car parks, acknowledging the logo.

Jumping Puddles

One night en route to a birth a fair distance from home, I received a frantic call that the baby was coming. I put my foot down along a deserted road in the outer suburbs with no other cars around at 2.30 am. With the moon full and high in the sky casting shadows along the road, I was on a mission to reach a woman birthing her sixth child that night. Suddenly, blue flashing lights appeared behind me – seemingly out of nowhere in the pitch-black night. As I pulled over, desperately wondering how I am going to get out of this one, I reach over to retrieve my licence from my bag, pressing the button to roll down the window and holding my licence out in anticipation. Meanwhile, my phone rings and as I press the green answer button on the dash, the police officer appears at my window. He beings to ask me the inevitable question when Bryan, the caller is on the line urgently stating, 'The baby is coming, I think she is ready, maybe pushing, and I haven't got the pool set up yet, how far away are you?' A loud roar fills the car speaker.

I smile brightly and look up at the policeman who is now almost in the car window listening to the sound emanating from the car speaker. 'What is that?' he asks in a loud whisper, as if she would hear him.

'I am a midwife, and I am on my way to help this woman give birth,' I pointed to the screen with her name on it and another loud roar with a piercing scream resonated from the speaker. 'Here's my licence, I'm aware I was speeding, but I really need to get to this woman.' I reach to turn the volume down slightly.

'Well, I really should give you a ticket, but I think you need to get to her. Do you need an escort?' I shake my head, still in shock, my heart racing. I thank him repeatedly, tossing my license onto the passenger seat as I prepare to put the car in gear. He leans back into my window, looking me straight in the eyes. 'Drive safe – please,' he says before turning and walking back to his car. The blue lights turn off, his car makes a U-turn, and the road is plunged into darkness.

Midwife Crisis

'Kel are you still there, what do I do?' Bryan inquired in a high-pitched panicked voice.

'I'll be there in 3 minutes,' I say pulling the car onto the dark road towards their house.

As I pulled up to their house, I seriously thought my heart would explode from my chest, the adrenaline in me was at an all-time high. I grabbed the oxygen tank, birth bag and literally ran into the house.

The family belonged to the Mormon community in Brisbane, having returned to Australia from the USA a few months earlier with their five other children. They aimed to live the simple life on a semi-rural property, growing vegetables and baking bread. All the children were home schooled, and they had no technical devices in their home, no smart phones, no television, no iPad. The eldest child was 10 and the youngest was 2 years old. Kaylee hailed from St Louis, an all-American girl and a former cheerleader, valedictorian, with a degree in sociology that she had never used. She had given up her other life when she met a handsome Aussie boy named Bryan, who initially came to their church as a young pastor. Upon arriving in Brisbane, the Mormon community set them up in a house with furniture, a car and a stocked pantry.

Kaylee was 30-weeks pregnant when they landed in Brisbane, and we had connected over Facebook during their transition to Australia. We planned the birth over FaceTime and finally met a few days after they settled into their immaculate home. The house was perfectly organised, adorned with bookshelves and family portraits on the walls. Each room had a crucifix and an altar for regular prayers. The children were exceptionally polite and well-mannered, offering tea and homemade scones during antenatal home visits. One visit I attended, they had picked me a bunch of wildflowers, wrapping them in newspaper and tying them with a ribbon.

Jumping Puddles

Kaylee spoke to the children with calmness, tenderness and a kindness, that displayed evident pride in them. The second eldest, Kieren, was fascinated with planes, aspiring to become a jet fighter pilot at the age of 8. While enjoying scones with fresh cream and homemade jam at their kitchen table, I heard the intricate details of a MIG 7, as he had memorised every detail. Visiting their home always made me feel like I was on the set of *Little House on the Prairie*. It was so very wholesome and there was this sense of calmness and warmth that filled me each time I visited.

On the night of her labour, Kaylee adorned herself in her birthing dress – a full-length, long-sleeved garment buttoned to the neck. She had shared the significance of the dress with me: it was a handmade creation by her grandmother, the very same dress she had worn for all of her births. Adhering to the principles of the Mormon religion, which discourages the exposure of flesh, Kaylee refrained from wearing clothes that revealed her arms and legs. Her skirts typically grazed her ankles and nothing she wore was tight fitting. The birthing dress, with its full coverage brought to mind the iconic black hooped dress worn by the character in *The Piano*.

By the time I had reached the house, navigating the long dimly lit corridor to the room at the end, I walked in on a scene that could have been out of a movie. Kaylee wearing her birthing dress, had stepped into the birth pool. It had only been partially inflated to one level. Stepping into the 20 cm or so of water lining the bottom of the pool, she squatted, the dress spilling over the sides of the pool and then completely submerging, dipping into the water at the front. With her hands on either side of the pool, she gripped the plastic tightly.

'The baby is coming,' she breathed out looking up at me, her face calm and blushed. She had only just noticed I was there. Women just know, their bodies work with them, their bodies and their babies work in unison. Watching this unfold in front of me is such a privilege and I have never taken this privilege for granted.

Midwife Crisis

'Okay, you do what you need to do,' I said as I placed my oxygen tank down but still had my bag on my back. In what seemed like slow motion, she gathered the front of the dress that was floating on the water with one hand, held onto the side of the pool with the other and then reached down to the puddle of water to bring her baby to her buttoned-up chest. He had not yet taken a breath, he wasn't really born into water, just on top of it. He began to stir as Kaylee blew in his face, his legs started to kick at her belly and he bobbed his head up and down, he let out an almighty cry and opened his eyes looking at his mother. She shushed him and gently eased herself onto her knees, holding him close to her face. He was covered in vernix – he was supposed to be at 42 weeks and 2 days.

I remembered I had my bag on my back just then. I put it down and sat down crossed legged next to the pool, watching her looking at her baby. She looked at me and smiled, radiating beauty. She looked up at Bryan and he laid a kiss on her lips that lingered longer than it should have in front of company, but it was one of those moments in time. He whispered he was sorry the pool wasn't filled, we all laughed and I told them we can claim this as a puddle birth.

This story brings to mind a similar birth experience when I left D alone at a party during the Christmas season. We had driven up to the Gold Coast to attends D's end of year work celebration. As was our usual practice, we drove separately. The event was formal, so I was dressed in a long green dress, heels and long glittery earrings. Naturally, I had my birth bag complete with equipment and a JIC bag (Just in Case) containing a change of clothes, spare undies, sneakers and a toothbrush for any unforeseen emergencies on my end.

The party kicked off and we were enjoying the company's catering and drinks (I of course was not drinking). I felt somewhat at ease that night and didn't have the feeling of being in my usual on call, on edge state. Uncharacteristically, I had left my phone in my handbag on a table for about 45 minutes. Normally, it is attached to my hand and is rarely put down. Heading to the bathroom I checked the phone to find five missed calls and three text messages from Mikki. Panic began to creep from my stomach. Please don't let this be her in labour, my mind kept repeating as I dialled her back.

'My waters have broken, and I think I'm in labour. Are you still at the party?' Mikki asked, breathing heavily as she picked up the phone on the first ring.

Mikki's first baby had been induced at 37 weeks due to pregnancy induced hypertension. Throughout this pregnancy she diligently monitored her blood pressure, and we implemented a regime of natural remedies to manage it. Mikki consistently reported feeling more relaxed and in tune with her body. Being allowed, to have control over it was vastly different to her previous care providers. Additionally, she had embarked on studying midwifery, which bolstered her confidence with newfound knowledge. Opting for a homebirth, Mikki aimed to minimise stress and increase her chances of experiencing a natural labour and birth.

During our last antenatal visit a few days prior, I informed Mikki that I had an upcoming function scheduled for the weekend she was due. However, I assured her of my availability to attend her birth and explained I would be on the Gold Coast but ready to travel to her. I also assured her that I would contact the second midwife to ensure she had additional support in case of any delays on my end. During our call, I asked her the usual standard questions, colour of water, baby movements, if she had pressure and how often the contractions were coming. She gave me the assurance that all was normal and that she wasn't ready to birth just yet, I'd likely have time to get back to Brisbane at this time of night. Despite that, I hurried back to D to tell him I had to go. He kissed me, told me to drive safe and not too fast, and to call when I arrived. I waved goodbye to the hosts and got in my car. The highway was clear and there was no roadworks to hold me up, thank goodness. Making it back to Brisbane within the hour was a smooth run.

Midwife Crisis

Arriving at Mikki's house I had to park a few houses away as there seemed to be a party going on in the street. Lugging my equipment from my car I realised I was in my green formal dress with the silver stilettos still on. There was no time to change, I grabbed my Converse sneakers, slipped off the stilettos at the last minute and hurried up the street barefoot.

The front porch light was on, but they always used the back door as the entry. I walked down the dark driveway, passing their bathroom window along the way. The light coming through the leadlight windows and the sound of a shower indicated that Mikki was in there. I could hear her emitting that low guttural moan that tells me labour is well established. Racing up the back steps, I dropped all the equipment I was carrying and moved to the bathroom.

'You didn't have to get so dressed up for me,' she said from the shower floor. She was leaning against the wall with the shower hose on her belly. She sat crossed legged and was naked. 'I wore my birth suit for you,' she said with a cheeky grin.

I pulled up the stool that her eldest son used to reach the toilet and sat down close to the shower door which was wide open. I leaned in to touch her knee. I always felt grounded when I touched them. It was a sign of connection, a sign that I was here and that she could let go now.

We chatted for a few minutes before the next wave took over her body. She moved to her hands and knees, and I took the shower head from her and aimed it at her back. The hot water sprayed out onto my dress, wetting my newly spray tanned legs and a stream of tan ran down my shin onto the white bathmat.

The sounds of James working in the kitchen to inflate the pool was reassuring. I had observed that it wasn't in the spot we initially designated for it when I arrived. Although it might be too late, I chose not to mention anything.

Jumping Puddles

Mikki expressed that she wanted to leave the shower, feeling dizzy and lightheaded from the heat. I turned off the shower and assisted her to her feet. As she stepped out, a stream of bright red blood trickled down her leg onto the bathmat, creating a small pool that mixed with the stain from my spray tan. I moved her to the lounge room and listened to her baby's nice rhythmic heartbeat resonating loudly from the doppler speakers. The presence of blood indicated that her cervix had likely dilated to its capacity, signalling that her body was ready. Although the pool was inflated to its capacity, there was little to no water in there. I motioned to James to hurry up with the water, and grabbing a large bucket from the laundry, he filled it and carried it to the pool. This probably added about 10 cm of water to the bottom. I didn't even get mad about the fact that the liner hadn't been fitted to the pool either.

Mikki stepped in. She stood for a bit waiting for the next contraction which built up the pressure she needed to prepare herself. James used this space to add in another half bucket of warmed water. Moving into a deep sumo squat, her hands went to the bottom of the pool to steady herself. Mikki roared with the wave that took over her body, her eyes closed tight, her mouth wide open. I grabbed my phone and flicked on the torch, her vagina parted, and a crinkled slither of a baby's head adorned with bright blonde hair was sitting there, waiting. The contraction stopped and Mikki panted and breathed out slowly and deeply. She began to push again, more of this blonde-headed babe emerged, this time with force to the brow line of the baby. James stood over her, his feet in the water, like being in a toddler's wading pool. He held her shoulders, and chanted 'Come on babe, you are doing it.'

Mikki's previous birth was intense and drawn out, resulting in a small baby with meconium aspiration, needing days of care in the special care nursery in a large tertiary hospital. She encountered breastfeeding issues and eventually bottle fed her baby formula. Determined to overcome her anxiety and fear, she had diligently worked with the support of counselling and my team at MAMA.

Midwife Crisis

She soon began to appear confident and trusting of her body and her ability to birth. She worked hard towards a normal intervention-free birth. James had initially been sceptical about having a baby at home, and voiced concerns about what the neighbours might think. During several planning session, I noticed that he would appear to shake when we discussed possible emergencies. It seemed as though he had absorbed all of Mikki's initial anxiety and fears of birth. Together, Mikki and I dedicated numerous hours to helping him gain confidence and prepare for their homebirth.

My second midwife had been texted when I was en route, and I had messaged her just as I was assisting Mikki out of the shower. I could hear her walking down the driveway now. She had informed the student midwife, and they had arrived together. I had momentarily forgotten about the student. They quietly appeared in the doorway of the kitchen. I gestured to them that the top of head was emerging into the very small amount of water that we had in the pool and waved the student over so that she could 'catch' this baby. I asked Mikki to lift her bottom slightly so that we could keep the baby above the water. With insufficient water for full submersion, it was decided to make it a land birth. As Mikki complied, the face of the baby slipped past her perineum. I guided the student's hand and placed it against it just as it tore. Fresh red blood dripped down her hand into the water, staining it pink. The baby continued to emerge, and within a second or two, the student held the baby's shoulders, his body slithering on to the towel I had placed over the small amount of water in the pool. Gurgling and attempting to cry, he was born at one minute past midnight.

The student held him above the puddle of water that had been in the pool, giving Mikki the chance to turn around to meet her baby. She sat in the pink water and took her baby into her arms. She tilted her head back and let out a wail. She had done it. The relief she experienced resonated through everyone it the room that night. The pool maintained a pleasing pink hue, the baby suckled at her breast from the minute he could get to her and I wasn't concerned about the blood loss. Her perineum would be sutured by us if necessary. I often employed an age-old midwife's technique of applying seaweed and manuka honey to small perineal tears. The seaweed aided in healing, while the honey minimised bacteria growth. I would diligently dress it daily for them in the postpartum days, utilising this incredible healing tool that I kept in my birthing bags for many years to come. I might have mended a perineum or two with my trusty seaweed and honey in a hospital setting as well. That night, I never changed out of that dress or removed my glittery earrings. I remained a barefoot, ball-gowned midwife, supporting a woman in achieving a much-needed healing birth, at home, in a puddle of water.

To be someone who cares deeply,
who suffers with others and for
others despite their own pain,
is to embody a rare strength.
It's showing kindness without
expecting it in return and being a
light in the darkest of places.

Chapter 9

Losing My Identity

Being a midwife is a defining aspect of my identity, setting me apart in a way that few professions do, perhaps only comparable to actors and sex workers who are often identified by the roles they play. This role has taken me to places and moments that most people never experience. I've witnessed women at their most raw and most vulnerable, offering support through tears, pain and screams. I've provided physical comfort by rubbing backs, arms and legs, applying hot packs to perineums and pressure points to toes. I have encouraged them to find their strength and push through the pain.

I've shared intimate moments, sitting on shower floors, holding knees apart during pushes on toilets, and even handling the less glamourous aspects of midwifery, like cleaning up poo and vomit. The nature of this job has led to experiences like being urinated on and occasionally bitten. I've assumed positions and performed procedures that diverge significantly from conventional jobs, such as putting my hands inside bodies and tending to engorged breasts. Being a midwife is more than a profession: it's a calling that many, including myself, take very seriously. It's a role that's challenging to switch off from, difficult to unwind after, and nearly impossible not to constantly contemplate. I found myself becoming obsessed, struggling to strike a balance and lacking separation between my work and personal life.

Returning home from a birth is always an adventure. Typically, I've just completed a 12 to 14-hour day, with minimal food, bathroom breaks or sips of water. Eagerly getting into my car, I crank the music, roll down the windows (even in the middle of winter) and navigate my way through the new bright, shiny day, trying to figure out what day of the week it might be. You lose track of time when the doors of the birth suite close behind you. I often drive on autopilot, following the same route, belting out familiar tunes to get me home. The drive home can be my reflection time, pondering what I could have done differently, or better. These thoughts can replay in my mind for days, especially after challenging births or those where I had to advocate strongly for the woman, or for myself.

The motivation behind writing this book is to share the journey of a midwifery career – and not just any midwifery career. It is about getting the story out there into the world, letting it unfold in all its complexity and perhaps offering support to other midwives who might undergo similar experiences, suffering similar traumas.

I don't possess a blueprint to make it easier for others, no magical strategies, or workshops, or a special pill to erase the pain. There is no treatment or specific support group for midwives like me. It's unfortunately something that gets bottled up inside, year after year, occasionally bubbling over, hitting like a wave before receding once again, to be hidden and covered up. It's invisible; a burden carried silently. It is intriguing how someone can appear normal externally, but internally, emotions churn and burn, waiting to resurface.

We must somehow redefine strength, recognise that true strength lies in the courage to discuss what's hurting us on the inside. There were times when I didn't even feel brave enough to talk about it – but now, here it is, in all its glory.

Losing My Identity

In the final weeks of my tenure in the hospital, my manager bestowed upon me the title of a 'rouge midwife' and questioned why I couldn't conform to the rules like the others. The label lingers in my thoughts, leaving a bitter taste. I haven't entirely embraced the title. I never intended to be a rouge midwife, and I don't believe I intentionally disregarded the rules to warrant such a label to be honest.

I aimed to provide women with choices for their birth, to empower them with knowledge about the full spectrum of childbirth. My commitment was to enable and educate women about their body's capability in giving birth. Additionally, I advocate for midwives to work within their full scope of practice. The core belief was that it is the woman's body and her baby, and therefore, it should be her choice. Forcing a woman to do something that she doesn't want to or dictating how she should experience childbirth contradicts the concept of empowerment to me. Knowledge, in this context, is power and the imbalance of power is evident when it comes to supporting birthing women. The hippocratic oath we take, stating that we do no harm, takes on a paradoxical meaning when we consider the growing incidence of birth violence and trauma. This is essentially where we do the most harm.

Birth trauma not only affects the birthing woman but also impacts the midwives who witness these traumatic events every day. I have spent years grappling and processing the events that changed my pathway, trying to understand how and why they occurred, and managing the shame associated with them. In the realm of midwifery, encountering unexpected outcomes is often considered a numbers game, a harsh reality that one may face during their career. Sadly, I experienced the loss of a baby under my care – an agonising event that deeply affected not only the parents of this baby, but also their midwife. Me.

The event that occurred has charted the course of my career and life ever since, a haunting presence day and night, profoundly shaping my identify as both a person, and more significantly, as a midwife.

Midwife Crisis

It is a burden that I carry with me, not by choice but by necessity. It shaped the way I practice, and it changed my appetite, in more ways than one, for risk. I feel compelled to bring it to the surface periodically, especially during recent job searches and interviews. On rare occasions, I recount the story, finding it challenging to get through, with the large lump that forms in my throat. Perhaps there's a need to vocalise it, a reminder that it was real and not just a nightmarish figment of my imagination. The desire to let it go persists, but the system's constraints, like shackles, prevent it. The experience looms over me like a large grey cloud, ready to burst, and my midwifery registration bears a conspicuous black mark.

I lie awake at night, pondering where it all went wrong and questioning how much longer I should dedicate myself to this profession that has inflicted so much pain. I am currently battling another challenge that has arisen against me because I cared, helped and supported a choice a woman made. My journey to this point is a rich and layered story, not a result of chance. I am not dangerous or reckless: I am considered and measured. I meticulously assess risks, rarely contemplating my own situation, instead focusing on others and what would benefit them. I often think that if I was to erase all of the mistakes I made, taken all the other paths I could have to get to where I am today, my story would look very different. It would only be removing the lines and the cracks that mark the voyage along the way.

I'm sharing this tale of this time, not as someone who had all the answers, but as one who lived courageously through it all, fought the battle, bore all the scars and survived the fight.

Chapter 10

The Shadows of Loss

The room was bathed in the warm glow of the early morning sun, a sharp contrast to the cold silence that had settled in like an uninvited guest. As a seasoned midwife, having been present at so many births in my 20-year career, nothing could have prepared me for this. The homebirth I had attended the previous night had ended in tragedy; the baby, despite the efforts of the paramedics and the second midwife, did not survive. It felt like it was all a dream, that it didn't really happen. I hadn't slept in 2 days now but yet I still had an undeniable energy that surged through my body.

I had always prided myself on my calm demeanour and unwavering confidence, qualities that had earned me the trust of countless parents. But now, I felt those very foundations shaking beneath me. The parents, a young couple full of dreams and love, had held their lifeless baby with a heartbreaking acceptance. They had not blamed me, their eyes filled with a sorrow so deep that it transcended words.

As I sat in the unusually quiet kitchen the following morning, I replayed the events in my mind, searching for the moment that I might have missed, the decision that could have made things different. My hands, still trembling from the shock, wrapped around a mug of untouched tea. I couldn't shake the feeling that I had failed, that my years of experience and intuition had somehow betrayed me. Why didn't my gut instinct, that I prided myself on time and time again, kick in?

Days turned into weeks, and the grief became a constant companion. I found myself withdrawing from my community, my family and my work which once was a comforting presence. I felt a ghostly shadow of my former self. I felt like I was in a fog, a strange deep fog, that had settled over me. My thoughts were jumbled, my mind raced and I couldn't shake the ache that sat on my chest. D & I attended the funeral, he wouldn't let me go alone. We drove to the service in silence, he knew I couldn't talk, knowing how badly broken I was. I remained in the car after we parked, breathing deeply and feeling numb. My eyes were fixed on the rows of headstones, the vibrant colours of flowers on the graves, and the mourners slowly making their way into the chapel. D tapped my hand and nodded, signalling it was time to go in. We entered the service after most of the guests had already been seated, standing at the back. D held my arm firmly, as if to keep me upright, while tears streamed down our faces. We listened to the chaplain conduct a service that should never have happened and watched as the parents laid their baby to rest. They had embraced me, whispering words of forgiveness and understanding, but it did little to lift the crushing weight of guilt I carried throughout that day and into the weeks, months and years that would follow.

It wasn't long before the regulatory board initiated an investigation. Homebirths, though legally supported, were always under scrutiny. The news of the baby's death spread quickly, and with it, a maelstrom of judgement and speculation. I was called to testify, to relive the harrowing night in excruciating detail. Every decision, every moment was dissected, analysed, and questioned. The investigation went on for months and it became constant burden to carry around with me. I didn't know from one day to the next if today was going to be the day that a decision was to be made, a decision that would determine my fate and the rest of my career.

The board's verdict came swiftly. While they acknowledged that I had followed protocol, offering choices and informed care and that I had done everything within my power, they deemed the risk too great. My license to provide homebirth services was revoked. I could still practise midwifery, but only within the confines of a hospital setting. The decision felt like a cruel twist of fate. I had chosen midwifery because of the personal, intimate care I could provide in the home environment, where women could make choices of their place of birth and their choice of care provider. Now, that chapter of my career was abruptly closed.

Losing the ability to conduct homebirths was more than just a professional setback; it was a personal devastation. My private practice, built on years of trust and dedication, began to crumble. Clients, seeking the homebirth experience, had to seek alternatives. Closing up my lifelong dream was a devasting blow, not only to me but to those that I employed, where the team I had created was like a family.

I found myself in an unfamiliar landscape, I was uncomfortable, I was fearful and I struggled to see myself and my passion for midwifery, stifled by the clinical confines of hospital walls. I wasn't ready for that, but yet I wasn't ready for my career to end just yet. I was conflicted, and ashamed as to where I had found myself.

Financial strains soon followed. Without the steady stream of homebirth clients from the clinic, my income dwindled. I had to let go of the MAMA Centre, a place that had been a sanctuary for so many women, midwives and myself. The empty office, once filled with the joyous cries of newborns and the laughter of mothers, now stood bare as a stark reminder of all I had gained, achieved and lost so quickly.

Midwife Crisis

Beyond the professional and financial toll, I struggled with a profound sense of shame. I avoided social gatherings, unable to face the whispered questions and sideways glances. I still have trouble answering the question of why I don't practice as a homebirth midwife, even still, after all these years. It profoundly breaks my heart and destroys my soul to say I lost a baby, that I lost someone's baby during a homebirth. Friends and colleagues reached out, offering support, but I found it hard to accept. I was always the carer, the caregiver and rarely was I on the receiving end. The shame was an insidious force, whispering in my ear, day in and day out, telling me I was unworthy of their kindness and words of compassion. It stung like a thousand bee stings.

Each night in that first year after, I would lie awake, the silence of the house deafening. Images of the baby's still form, as I held them in my bloodied hands and the tiny coffin that I had watched being lowered into the ground, haunted my dreams. They were constant reminders of my perceived failure. I tried therapy sessions which provided some relief, to just talk it out and to be allowed to feel the shame and guilt, to say it out loud. But the road to healing was long and fraught with setbacks.

I knew I had to confront the demons, to forgive myself, but it was easier said than done.

In time, I began to see glimpses of hope. I turned to teaching, sharing my passion with cohorts of young and fresh midwives. It was difficult place to be in the beginning. I struggled to turn off the independent midwife in me, it wasn't ever going to be the same as private practice, but it was a way to reconnect with my passion for midwifery. I was scared, frightened I would fail at this too somehow but the gratitude of the students and the women I helped and supported provided the balm I needed to apply to my very wounded spirit.

Slowly, I started to rebuild my life, finding a new balance and a new way to cope. The pain of losing the baby and my practice has never fully disappeared, but it became a part of the story, a chapter that taught me resilience and the capacity to endure.

My journey through grief and shame is a testament to the strength of the human spirit. I learned to navigate the shadows of loss, finding a way to honour the memory of the baby while forging a new path forward. It was not the life I had envisioned, and my dreams were much bigger than this, but it was one filled with purpose and renewed determination to make a difference, one birth at a time.

Lost and yearning for the person I once was, I now strive to protect the person I've become and nurture the person I deserve to be.

Chapter 11

Storm Warning

You're never given a warning about a notification until it is officially received by the regulatory board. There are no formal processes to anticipate the submission of a report, usually initiated by hospital managers or administrators following incidents, whether minor or major. In most circumstances, you are given 2 weeks to respond to the accusations. It's like a hurricane approaching, but without the storm warning signals.

It was like any other day in early December of 2016. Everyone was getting ready for the Christmas break, school holidays had just begun and the heat in Brisbane was unbearable as it usually was at that time of year. The bookings had reduced during the month as we wanted the staff to have a much-needed break, so between two midwives we would share the on-call duties. The other practitioners would take a break during the holidays, so the clinic was closed for the first time since we had opened. It meant that I would be able to have some time off from admin to do regular activities. It was never far from my mind. I attempted to do normal everyday things, to keep my mind and body at a pace I could manage without falling into a deep hole. I recall I was at the hairdressers when I received the call from a representative at the regulatory board. They informed me that they had received three notifications about my practice. One involved the loss of the homebirth baby, while the other two completely blindsided me. I couldn't understand why I would be reported for those, knowing that they had turned out to be births that I had transferred into the hospitals for care. In that moment, the world seemed to come to a standstill. The representative explained where the complaints had originated from, assuring me that I would receive the full details in the mail in the coming days.

Waiting for those details seemed like an eternity, even though it was only a matter of days. I was engulfed by fear and the uncertainty of what it all meant. Unsure of where to turn or who to talk to, I quickly resorted to googling what to do when you receive a notification from the regulatory board. The advice from all opinions was to seek support from the Nursing and Midwifery Union, and I reached out to them as quickly as I could. They provided me with valuable advice and information. I was told to make a statement and to gather all the information and any documents I had regarding the notifications. It felt so robotic and mechanical, but I went along with it and prepared what I could. Additionally, they offered me the opportunity to speak with a lawyer who worked pro bono with the Queensland Nursing Union. At first, I misunderstood what this meant and felt as though I was trapped somehow. Would I really need a lawyer?

When I spoke with the lawyer over the phone, she was direct in her reasoning why I needed her and assured me that she was on my side and planned to support me in the investigation all the way. I promptly accepted the advice she gave and scheduled a meeting with her for the following day, where she would prepare me for the formal notification from the regulatory board.

The notification arrived via email at first, then followed by official correspondence in the mail. The lawyer worked tirelessly and diligently, proving various aspects to be inaccurate. We continued to work together for over a year on the report.

Storm Warning

As I was still harbouring underlying grief, trauma and stress in the weeks following the stillbirth, I found it increasingly difficult to maintain focus. Reading over the notifications increased my anxiety and I was constantly on edge. The words on the pages seem to glare at me, pointing out all my faults. Yet I was often drawn back to them, maybe to check that it was real. My stomach would burn, acid creeping its way up into my throat that sat there for days and weeks. I lay in bed at night desperately wanting sleep to take it all away, but it never did. I tried to keep busy, attempting to never be alone with my thoughts. The words on the notifications haunted me, judged me, damned me. I began to panic. My nerves were frayed, and I experienced bouts of severe anxiety. I broke down frequently, usually alone and not within ear shot or eyesight of anyone else. On the outside, I still looked the same – I had to, for everyone's sake – but inside, I was in an acute state of disaster. The notifications remained my own private burden, a secret that gnawed at me incessantly, consuming my thoughts every minute of every hour.

My confidence was shattered. I lacked faith or trust in myself or the women I was caring for, even though they had been well prepared for birth, and I had provided them with the best opportunity for a natural, normal birth. I just couldn't trust it. In the months that followed the notifications, I asked the other midwives in the team to take over as primary midwives for the women I was caring for. I worked as the back-up midwife and took a major step back. I sat on the peripheral, watching from afar as it felt safer for me, for everyone. I buried myself in administration tasks or cleaning the clinic, anything to take me off the clinical side of the job. I would spend hours photocopying notes and preparing statements for the lawyer well into the night when all the staff had gone home. I often came home exhausted as if I had been at births, but it wasn't the same euphoric exhaustion I would get from witnessing birth. It was a deep sense of depletion. Cortisol levels surged through me every minute of the day along with a deep sense of humiliation and shame.

Midwife Crisis

My practice had not been suspended or restricted during the course of the investigation – it continued over a harrowing 12 months, between the back and forth with lawyers, the regulatory board and the union. It soon took its toll on me. I couldn't continue to practise without knowing what was going to happen next. There was a real fear that my registration could be cancelled or restricted in some way, even though my lawyer was confident that this wouldn't occur. My practice underwent dramatic changes, and I made the difficult decision to cease practice and close the businesses. I began the arduous task of releasing staff from their contracts, moving women into other services and care providers and endured the process of selling and giving away the furniture and fittings of my beautiful MAMA Centre. I was fragile and frightened but never acknowledged it as I set about doing the tasks that needed to be done.

Enduring countless months of agony and engaging in extensive discussions with my lawyer, I eventually acquiesced to a registration undertaking that barred me from conducting homebirths. Additionally, the regulatory board mandated that I complete a course focused on ethical decision-making in healthcare practice. Needless to say, this was a significant blow to my pride, leaving me feeling utterly defeated and overwhelmed with guilt.

With each passing day, a profound sense of emptiness grew within me. I chose to shield my extended family from the turmoil I was experiencing, as it dawned on me how my profession made my parents and other members of my family proud. Proud of my achievements and how special it was, to be a midwife. I couldn't face telling them I had failed at this. Although my midwifery and allied health team provided unwavering support, I couldn't shake the guilt of letting them down and shattering their aspirations. My own dreams lay shattered and fragmented into countless pieces. The day I gathered my team and announced the closure of the MAMA Centre is etched into my memory, a painful reminder of what we had built together. Despite my best efforts to maintain composure, the anguish was palpable as I confessed that I could no longer sustain the remarkable service we had all poured our hearts and souls into.

Every day, even now as I write this, I grapple with the harsh truth that a woman is without her baby in her arms. I lost an extraordinary business and am left with nothing but the memories, which remain vividly etched in my mind. Frequently, I am reminded of that event, especially when I write the biannual compliance report to the board, assuring them that I no longer attend homebirths as a midwife, I document my current workplace and my role there. What is not documented are the many sleepless nights spent reflecting on the entire ordeal.

Midwife
{mid wy-fe} noun

The masters of keeping calm in a
crisis while at the same time
providing self-belief, support,
empowerment, advice, counsel
and guidance to the women they
care for, all the while delivering their
babies.
This is the definition
of a superhero.

Unknown

Chapter 12

Midwife – It's a Verb

At my 50th birthday party, my eldest son, Luis, delivered a heartfelt speech, recounting a moment in a meeting with male advertising executives. When he proposed a solution to a problem that was under discussion, his boss dismissively remarked. 'We're not saving babies here Luis.' In response, Luis proudly asserts that he knows someone who does save babies every day and expressed his deep pride for me. This touching speech moved me so much, recognising the impact I have had on my children in the years I have practised as midwife. His recognition of the significance of my job in saving lives every day speaks volumes.

Saving babies is ingrained in our core responsibilities as midwives. Every dedicated midwife can share stories of successful interventions that have preserved and nurtured life. However, the weight of our profession also carries the burden of the one we couldn't save. In critical moments, our training kicks in, urging us to act swiftly and decisively. We possess the skills to assist a newborn in breathing, utilising equipment and medications when needed. Yet, there is an essence of our practice that lies in the profound recognition that keeping the baby close to their mother can be a lifeline in itself.

Midwife Crisis

First-time parents considering a homebirth often enquire about the emergency equipment available. A homebirth midwife, akin to a boy scout, is always prepared.

We carry an array of equipment that can be used for emergency situations including an oxygen cylinder, a bag and mask, oxygen tubing, postpartum drugs such as syntocinon, syntometrium and mistoprosal. We have IV fluids, IV lines, IV cannulas, cord clamps and more. However, one unique addition to our emergency toolkit is breadboards. They have proven invaluable in various scenarios and have even played a role in saving a life.

In one situation, a baby born at home in water required additional oxygen support. We were equipped with oxygen tanks and infant masks and understood the importance of delayed cord clamping in home births. Therefore, we often refrain from immediately clamping or cutting the umbilical cord after birth, keeping the mother and baby connected. In this instance, we needed to provide extra oxygen to the baby in the birth pool without separating them from their mother. As the umbilical cord continued to pulsate, supplying oxygen rich blood to the baby, we improvised by finding a large breadboard in the kitchen. We floated the board in the water, placed the baby on it, and ensured that the board was partially submerged. This allowed the baby to remain close to their mother, while receiving the appropriate flow of oxygen, staying warm with a wet hand towel and a layer of warm water covering them. This arrangement facilitated better access to the baby's airway and ensured the correct direction of oxygen flow. In these situations, you do what needs to be done. The baby pinked up, flexed arms and legs and soon was back with their mother.

Recognising the usefulness of this trick, I purchased six large breadboards to keep on hand in our equipment boxes. They came in handy not just for emergencies but also for providing support during suturing for small perineal tears. By slipping them between mattresses and bed bases, they acted like stirrups however much less clinical. Additionally, head torches were added to our equipment bags, always a handy tool for those nights in darkened rooms when you need two hands. It saved us from switching on bright overhead lights and disturbing the ambiance and peacefulness of the room.

Working as a midwife in hospitals can be either fulfilling or soul-destroying, depending on the time, place and institutional culture. In my early career, fresh out of university with just a year of experience, I worked at a small private hospital in a coastal town. I was fortunate and confident enough to walk into the hospital and ask for a job, and surprisingly I was welcomed with open arms. This hospital was well-known in the area as a supportive, woman-centred facility. It was favoured by the affluent residents of the coast.

It was there that I learned about water birth and worked alongside some of the most incredible midwives and obstetricians I have ever met. I learned from the best. One obstetrician, in the early years of private practice, particularly stood out. This individual has since made significant contributions to women-centred obstetric care and CTG monitoring.

I remember working as the midwife for one of their private patients. The woman, in the birth pool, began to push, and as usual, the OB was called in to catch the baby. However, as the baby began to emerge, the OB just sat beside me, watching without moving. I gently elbowed them, indicating that the baby needed guidance, but they shook their head, signalling that I should be the one to catch the baby.

While we silently communicated through hand signals, the baby was born and floated to the surface. I set down the torch I was holding, scooped up the baby, and handed it to the proud mother. The doctor sat cross-legged on the bathroom floor, amazed. Later that night, as we filled out paperwork at the birth suite desk, I gently asked why they hadn't picked up the baby. Sheepishly, they admitted that they had never seen a water birth or caught a baby in water before and were unsure of what to do. They thanked me for being there that night and for not making them look foolish.

Years later, I sat in the audience of a conference where they were a guest speaker. During their speech, they recalled that birth and the lessons they had learned from a midwife. Feeling very humble, I blushed and gave them a small wave from my seat. We ran into each other later at the conference, laughing and chatting about that unforgettable night. They admitted that the memory had been etched into their mind and confided that they wished they had become a midwife instead of a doctor. They expressed eternal gratitude for all that midwives had taught them over the years and for the collaboration they had enjoyed with midwives throughout their career.

Then of course there is the flip side of working as a midwife in large institutions, where being a midwife often feels more like navigating a medieval battlefield than a collaboration amongst 21st century healthcare professionals, each having their own area of expertise. I encountered Ellie during my tenure in a hospital. An intelligent, independent, career-oriented and seriously vivacious woman, she struggled with significant anxiety about impending motherhood. Her nervousness often reached palpable levels during our 20-minute clinic visits. Our discussions frequently revolved around her myriad of concerns, ranging from the type of mattress in her baby's cot to the choice of skin lotion she could use in pregnancy. Our clinic appointments, however, were always enjoyable, filled with laughter, and marked by a sense of trust and a strong bond between us.

Unfortunately, Ellie's pregnancy coincided with the strict lockdowns which meant that partners were not permitted to accompany women to the clinic appointments. This added an extra layer of anxiety for some, especially for those experiencing pregnancy for the first time. The absence of partners meant they couldn't share the joys of hearing their baby's heartbeat or witnessing ultrasounds together. Some women even required special permits to leave home for antenatal care, and access to the hospital was limited to childbirth only. The prospect of partners being disallowed from labour and birth, although it didn't materialise in Australia, added an extra layer of stress to an already challenging situation for the women, their families and midwives during that time.

Ellie and I formed a strong connection, and I met Drew, her husband, via FaceTime first, then in person towards the latter stages of pregnancy. They were both filled with excitement and had learned hypnobirthing techniques they planned to implement during labour and birth. Ellie aimed to labour at home and then come to the hospital when she felt she was ready. She had gained confidence and trusted her body by this stage.

As with all well-made plans, this one did not unfold as expected. Ellie reached 41 weeks and 4 days, a journey marked by a substantial amount of anxiety, stress, a few false starts and ultimately reluctantly succumbing to the system's pressure to undergo induction of labour. I was not a supporter of the induction plan for Ellie, but, as is often the case, the system prevailed. The ominous words from doctors about potential risks to the baby typically leads parents to agree. We set a date and devised a plan. My midwife colleague began the induction at 7 am and cared for Ellie and Drew until their labour had established. An established labour was typically determined by the frequency, intensity and regularity of contractions, along with the progress of cervical dilatation. Ellie's labour was progressing well, and she had been in established labour for a few hours. Despite her fatigue, Ellie remained cheerful but sought further pain relief. She had already attempted various non-medicalised methods, such as using the shower spray jets to alleviate her back pain, utilising her TENS machine, and trying gas without success. Now, she deliberated whether to opt for an epidural, carefully weighing up the pros and cons of this form of pain relief in her characteristic thoughtful manner.

I assumed responsibility for her care around 7 pm and would support her through the night. She eventually requested an epidural, a deviation from her original birth plan. However, it proved beneficial in helping her relax and get some much-needed rest after an exceptionally long and challenging day. In the latter stages of the labour, with three doctors present, the narrative shifted abruptly from tranquillity to chaos, rendering the soothing elements of fairy lights, hypnobirthing tracks and essential oils ineffective.

Ellie faced a given timeframe to push her baby out, with the looming threat of an instrumental birth or a caesarean section echoing loudly from all three of the doctors in the room. Politely refusing the C-section, Ellie sought clarification on the instruments mentioned and, rightfully so, requested a full explanation for the suggested interventions. One of the doctors, in my opinion, unnecessarily introduced some degree of hysteria, stating that it had been a long day, and that it would be best to 'deliver' the baby sooner rather than later. Ellie once again asked for additional time to continue pushing, supported by her husband's plea for a calmer approach from the doctors. He even expressed a desire to have a private discussion with his wife and me, their midwife. Unfortunately, all these requests were denied by the team, who maintained a stern, arms crossed stance in the room.

Even though I had been Ellie's midwife for her whole pregnancy I was considered completely redundant in the current situation. Despite my attempts to communicate with the senior OB, she dismissed me, taking on the position of leader and seemingly knowing what was best for Ellie at the time. After some painstaking discussions, Ellie agreed for the instrumental birth, with the condition that they would consult her with the process. As quickly as she agreed, the stirrups were put up and her legs placed in them.

The baby had not yet crowned. All three doctors centred around Ellie's raised stirrup legs, her lower half of her body completely exposed and visible for all that were in the room to see. All three of the doctors concurred after each of them had done a vaginal examination – one after another, that the baby was in an OP position meaning that the baby was facing the wrong way up. They planned to use the forceps to help turn the baby as it came down. Ellie was instructed to push by the doctor, who stood between her legs wielding the forceps, and as she begun the doctor placed one blade inside of her vagina. A piercing scream came from Ellie and she jumped backwards – even though her legs were in the stirrups her body had completed moved up the bed. The doctor preparing to insert the other blade, stopped and asked Ellie to return to the assigned position in the stirrups.

'Seems like your epidural isn't as dense as I had hoped,' she said, 'we can top that up and I'll add some lignocaine to your peri, that should take care of it.'

By this stage Ellie was panicked, crying hysterically, and requesting them to stop. The second blade was placed and then locked into position to begin the task of bringing the baby towards the perineum. Ellies scream of intense pain and fear was evident, which still did not stop the process. Drew and I were at her head, trying to keep her calm and asking her to focus on us. She was shaking uncontrollably and sobbing. 'Take it out of me, please stop, please stop,' she said over and over again. I glanced at the CTG monitor, the baby's heart rate was within normal and reactive, Ellie was still having contractions, that were within normal range. It appeared to me that there was time. I moved to the end of the bed where the doctor was. Over the top of Ellie's leg, I asked if she could just stop for a minute.

Ignoring my request, she received a pair of scissors from her colleague standing beside her. She did not take her eyes of the perineum. Wondering if she heard me, I asked again. I am sure she heard me, I am sure she understood what I asked her to do. The doctors were wearing clear plastic face shields which reflected like mirrors. A moment later I watched as her scissors sliced through Ellie's perineum, the sound of cutting flesh still rings in my ears. The blood began to gush, her vagina gaping wide open, flesh and muscle visible. The forceps were pulled one more time and the baby was dragged out of Ellie's body, with the steel blades still attached to his head. A warm baby blanket was placed in my hands by someone else in the room, this was the receiving blanket and once the blades were removed, a very stunned, swollen-headed baby landed in the blanket I automatically held out. I felt numb, I was stunned at what I had just witnessed, I looked at this baby that was screaming in my arms, bloodied and bruised, I took the baby and placed him on Ellie's chest. Ellie by this stage was hyperventilating, sobbing and shaking. I was silently doing the same.

The blood continued to pour from the open wound. It was pooling in the bucket and spilling over. With the numerous individuals in the room, someone must have pressed the emergency buzzer, initiating a code pink. More medical staff rushed to the room amplifying the chaos and confusion. There was a notable absence of the usual order and system seen during emergency situations. It seemed unusually out of control. Ellie was now experiencing a severe haemorrhage and the obstetrician was still endeavouring to extract her placenta. I glanced down and noticed that the doctor was wearing white gum boots; there were splatters of blood across the toes. Ellie asked me to take the baby off her, she was shaking too violently to hold him securely. I gently took him from Ellie's chest, wrapped the blanket tighter around him and held him for Drew to see, all the while keeping an eye on what was unfolding between Ellie's legs. The baby began crying loudly, signalling he had coped well during his dramatic entry into the world. There was a flurry of activity as the paediatricians departed, realising their services were no longer required. Midwives who had arrived with them packed up and left, while the remaining staff continued to address the haemorrhage. One of the paediatricians had looked him over before they left and commented that he will have some bruising and a headache for a few more days, adding that he looked like a tough kid.

Ellie was weak, blankly staring at the ceiling and trying to control her breathing. She held on to Drew's hand so tightly I could see her knuckles turning white. I continued to hold their baby close to my chest to keep him warm and comforted.

Inspecting the perineum for damage and attempting to stem the blood flow, the same doctor that had facilitated the birth, announced condescendingly that Ellie had sustained a third-degree tear, like Ellie had done that to herself. She asked for another doctor's opinion, the two of them inspecting Ellie's vagina and perineum like they were mechanics inspecting an engine in a car. They began making calls to the theatre. Ellie would need a repair under a general anaesthetic. With the bleeding still uncontrolled, a large piece of gauze was placed into Ellie's vagina to stem the blood loss. I now had to prep her for theatre. The room had been vacated of all the medical staff other than one of the junior doctors, who was attempting to get Ellie to sign a consent form for surgery, asking questions regarding allergies and medications. Ellie continued to stare at the ceiling, still in a dazed state of shock and vaguely answered yes and no to each respective question on the list.

We moved to the theatre quickly with the help of a wardsman. Ellie was wheeled directly to the OT. She was shivering under the thin waffle blanket, wildly looking around the cold clinical room. I hardly recognised this woman. The confident, prepared and bold woman that I had met, was gone. She looked up at me from the trolley as we prepared to move her to the theatre bed. Her eyes were so big, her face pale, she looked like a small version of herself.

'Is the baby, okay?' she asked as she was lifted onto the bed by a team of theatre staff. I held her hand until her arms were taken from me to be tethered to the BP cuff and the drip. Her legs were placed into yet another pair of stirrups and the anaesthetic doctor leaned over her, giving her instructions that she was to count backwards from ten as the anaesthesia began to take effect. I watched her eyes roll back and close as she mouthed the number eight.

Midwife Crisis

I had left Drew in the birth room with his newborn son. Another night that the ward was short staffed, and I had asked another midwife to watch over them while I escorted Ellie to the operating theatre. When I walked back into the birth suite room, there was no other midwife present. Drew was alone, cradling his newborn son in his arms, staring into his eyes. He had been crying and he wiped the newest tears away out of embarrassment when I walked in. The room looked like a war zone. Amid the rush to get Ellie to the theatre on the birthing bed, the wheels of the bed inadvertently passed through a pool of thick, viscous blood, leaving tracks that stretched from the door to the centre of the room. These stark tracks underscored the recent trauma that had unfolded within these walls. The room bore the aftermath of a hectic medicalised birth: packaging strewn about, IV fluid lines trailing, towels and baby blankets scattered, and discarded syringes littering the floor. At the back, the resuscitation cot remained pushed against the wall behind the green privacy curtain, blood splatters staining its surface. It was difficult to assess whether it was fresh or old, adding to the unsettling atmosphere of the room.

'Are you okay?' I whispered to Drew as I approached him, I placed my hand on his shoulder, peering over to check out the baby. The little boy tightly wrapped in the hospital bunny rug had a frown on his face, and likely a bad headache from the look of those marks, which had now turned a bright red colour. He had a lump on the side of his skull about the size of a 50-cent piece and one of his eyes was swollen shut, the other one looking at Drew. 'What a way to come into the world, little man. I'm so sorry,' I whispered to him, running my finger down his velvety soft cheek.

'What the fuck happened, Kel?' Drew said looking directly at me, searching for an explanation, he spoke quickly and like he couldn't get it all out fast enough. 'Is she okay, is he okay, what the fuck just happened?' he shook his head, taking a seat on the chair that he had been assigned to use after the chaos that was his son's birth.

Midwife – It's a Verb

'I don't know. I'm so sorry, she is going to be okay. She had a big tear and they are stitching it up, they have had to give her a GA to put her to sleep. She lost a lot of blood.' The words rolled off my tongue slowly so he could take it all in. I looked around the room, acknowledging this clean-up was all mine to manage.

I picked up a plastic bin, lined with a yellow hazardous waste liner and carried it around the room with me, putting everything on the floor into it. I picked up the bloodied towels and the cannulas that still had blood in them, the IV lines and leftover half bags of fluid from the IV poles. I picked up the bed sheets that had been covered in her blood and discarded to the floor, filling the laundry skip with red stained sheets. I noticed that the scrub shirt I had on had patches of Ellie's blood on it too. My wrists, where the gloves didn't reach, were streaked with blood. I went to the sink, removing the gloves I had worn for a few hours now, my hands sweaty and itchy. I began to wash vigorously at my arms and my hands. I took off my scrub shirt, which I had slipped over my own clothes before going to theatre and discarded it with the rest of the linen. Her blood was everywhere and on everything.

Drew let out a sigh and stood up still holding onto the baby in his arms – he was a large man, tall and solid. I felt tiny in his presence. He moved effortlessly with the baby in his arms, unlike some new dads who were scared to even move a muscle when they held their newborn for the first time. Drew walked over to the resus cot and gingerly put him down, I switched on the overhead heater as I passed by with yet another bloodied towel and Drew just stood there, looking at him, inspecting his son's tiny fingers. He ran is own calloused fingers gently over the marks on his face.

'Do you think these will be permanent?' He asked me, his voice low and gentle.

Knowing that they would fade, I came over and stood beside him.

Midwife Crisis

'They will eventually fade but they might be there for a few weeks. And this lump on his head will go down soon too,' I said, cupping my hand gently over the lump on the baby's head. He was now asleep under the heater. He looked so peaceful and totally unaware of all that his mother had endured for him.

'Drew, I am so sorry, I couldn't stop her, I tried, and I asked her to stop ...' I felt the hot tears well up. They began to fall and I didn't wipe them away.

I felt so powerless, so out of control and so responsible all at once. Every time something like this occurs, it pains me deeply. I find myself struggling to provide explanations and defend the actions of a system that has caused such damage, damage that will take a long time to heal. This birth was brutal and so far from normal. I often questioned whether I was the only one who felt this sense of responsibility, wondering if I had failed the women by being a part of it.

I spent weeks with Ellie and Drew, debriefing, deconstructing the labour and birth and purely giving support. She was damaged. Many times, I sat with her in her lounge room during our postnatal visits, witnessing her break down and the overwhelming devastation of what happened to her. It was rare to see her smile or to hear that she was doing okay, because, in truth, she wasn't okay at all. She was damaged mentally, emotionally and physically. Her perineum was a jagged mess, she couldn't walk without pain and a throbbing feeling for many months afterwards. Despite seeking help from various support services including a physiotherapist, specialised perineal doctors, obstetricians and gynaecological specialists, all of whom assured her that she would heal, Ellie's condition did not improve.

She sought treatment from a psychoanalyst for trauma but remained deeply broken. She struggled to believe that she would ever enjoy sex again and faced many challenges with bonding and feeding her baby. This ordeal led her into a deep depression that lasted for many months. I maintained close contact with her, seeing her regularly, and our relationship evolved into a friendship that I still cherish today. Her unwavering trust in me surpassed anything I could have imagined, especially considering how deeply she had been affected by what she had endured.

My own trauma from her birth consumed much of my thoughts and emotions. I often found myself dwelling on what I could have done differently, whether I should have spoken up sooner, or somehow intervened to prevent what happened to her. While I knew I couldn't turn back time, there were countless moments when I wished I could.

It was a genuine surprise when Ellie called me almost 2 years later, announcing that she was pregnant again. My initial reaction was one of shock, and I even questioned whether she felt truly ready. Both physically and mentally, her scars had barely healed, considering all that she had been through. Our conversation that day delved extensively into her past and some experiences that she had dealt with through recent therapy, her journey to recovery and her newfound hope for a different birth experience. I was so honoured that she had chosen me to support her again. That level of trust is truly invaluable. Throughout her entire pregnancy, we worked closely together. Ellie appeared focused and well prepared. She was clear about her preferences and had a plan in place. Having moved an hour away from the hospital during this pregnancy, Ellie and Drew devised back up arrangements for a closer hospital to take them if her labour progressed quickly. I committed to being there for her, irrespective of my schedule, even if it meant skipping a day off. My commitment to Ellie and Drew was unwavering.

One day, not long before Ellie's labour began, I was met in the hallway of the birth suite by one of the hospital's senior obstetricians. He was often described as a gentle giant, standing at 6 foot 3 or so, with a spray of wild salt and pepper hair that looked like it needed a good brush. I heard my name called out in his loud booming voice. It was always a surprise that he even knew the names of the midwives. Knowing well in advance who it was, I turned on my heels and watched him walking his off kilter walk towards me, in blue scrubs, orange duck bill mask not quite fixed on his face correctly, with a posse of student doctors behind him who were all trying to keep up with him. He was seemingly on a mission, in full stride.

'Make sure you cut an episiotomy on that previous 3rd degree tear of yours coming up, won't you?' He said pointing a long finger at me as he came closer. I was stopped still, all 5 foot 2 of me in heels. I knew he was talking about Ellie. He wouldn't know her name but would have read her file recently.

'Umm, I'm not sure she is going to need an episiotomy Doctor, I'm pretty good at keeping them intact, and we have done a lot of work on that peri,' I said nervously smiling my biggest smile.

'I am sure you are, but I don't want to see her in OT again, so best cut one,' he boomed at me as he strode past, so fast he nearly knocked me over. The posse of student OBs all looked at me quizzingly and I may have caught one whispering 'as if' under their breath.

I had no intention of cutting a routine episiotomy on Ellie. If it was warranted at the time, I would consider it. The hospital had recently introduced a policy aimed at reducing the occurrence of third- and fourth-degree tears, which recommended cutting episiotomies early and routinely. Ellie and I had discussed this, and her preference was to tear naturally rather than to incur another episiotomy that had the potential to extend. She was willing to take the risk. This was her birth and her body this time around. I was crossing every finger and every toe hoping and praying she didn't tear.

On a hot summer night in early December, the call came from Ellie. Her labour had started naturally, she was somewhat in denial but after talking for a few minutes, and recognising the signs of labour becoming established, I encouraged her to start making her way into the hospital. It took some time for me to convince her that it was indeed labour. I began preparing for my own trek to the hospital.

It was now reaching peak hour on a weekday, so I would be navigating unpredictable traffic from my side of town to the hospital. What would normally be a 30-minute drive could turn into an hour as I needed to cross the city through a heavily congested route. Making the drive at this time of the day was typically filled with heightened anxiety for me, triggered by the smallest delays, such as waiting for the elevator on my floor. I opted for the stairs, providing a faster descent to my own car park. The constant stop-start traffic annoyed me. Listening to a podcast to distract me often helped, but today I was inundated with thoughts of the what-ifs. *Would I arrive in time? Would they? What if she gave birth in the car? What if the baby was in distress? Was the baby okay? Had her waters broken since I last spoke to her? What if there is meconium?* These irrational thoughts persisted throughout the journey, and I yearned to reach the hospital to ease my concerns.

As I neared the hospital's driveway, I received a text from them to say they were still 15 minutes away. I noticed a subtle release of tension in my shoulders. I opted for the stairs again, this time from the car park, pushing myself to ensure that I reached the birth suite before them.

Walking into the birth suite that night my heart beat a little faster. This was becoming more common. Why was I so anxious? Maybe it was to be my perpetual state. As I pushed the double doors open, I slowed my breath, reminding myself to ease into it, be calm, stay focused, and not to let the trauma of her last birth rattle me. *This birth was going to be different*. I repeated this little mantra over and over again to myself, trying to steady my nerves. Reporting to the unit manager of the birth suite that night, I informed her of Ellie's imminent arrival and current condition. As the manager began to express her concerns about Ellie's past history, I acknowledged them, but remained composed. My priority was to create a safe and comforting space for Ellie's arrival.

Midwife Crisis

I gained a reputation for meticulously preparing a birth room, and it was during this preparation time that I felt most calm and relaxed. My birth bag was akin to Mary Poppins' carpet bag – seemingly bottomless. From fairy lights and diffusers to essential oils, doppler and pinards, a TENS machine, lollipops, snacks, socks, headphones and a portable speaker, you name it, I had it. If needed, I could transform a room within minutes.

With the diffuser on, the lights turned to a hue of blue and green, the Spotify birth track playing, and the necessary medical equipment checked and neatly tucked away out of sight, I started to relax. Taking a moment to look around, I felt proud of the safe space I had created, contributing to a serene and comforting atmosphere. Sometimes, small changes can bring a touch of warmth and comfort to the clinical setting of a birth suite room.

When Ellie and Drew arrived, they were in the full swing of labour. She smiled her big bright smile at me as she held on to the doorframe as she entered the birth room, riding the wave of yet another contraction. She was concentrating, her head down and her body just following the lead. She had her AirPods in and eyes closed as the contraction hit its peak, the smile and brightness disappeared, and her forehead crinkled and furrowed. Her breathing paced and she exhaled deeply. Inhaled through her nose and exhaled again. She was doing the J breath, a technique in breathwork that helps focus the direction of the breath in a J motion, in and out, down and up.

I stood looking at this woman, this woman who was so in control and leaving her body to do the work, opposed to her mind. Meanwhile, Drew was madly unpacking, moving quickly and with purpose. He isn't a small man, he always seemed so clumsy and had a loud booming voice. I adored him to be honest, his boyish charm and innocence was somewhat comical. Unpacking he was making so much noise, asking Ellie where he should put things, not necessarily understanding she was deep in her zone. Not watching where he was going, he tripped over a stainless-steel bucket that I had moved out of his way once but missed the second time. It caused a deafening noise, as it spun on its edge and landed on its side.

Ellie sharply looked up and gave him a look that could kill, but immediately put her head back down, taken over by another contraction – I stepped over to where he stood frozen, looking at me as I laid my hand on his arm. Picking up the bucket with the other hand, I kept hold of both of them for safety reasons. I gently rubbed his upper arm, he understood – he stopped, stood and turned to look at Ellie. She was riding yet another furious wave. I heard him mimic her breathing patterns, he looked at me, went to say something but stopped short. I nodded and guided him towards her. He helped her move into the room, I closed the door and the curtain behind them. They were safe now in this space, that was just us. The room was silent other than the music softly coming from the small speaker, I didn't want to break the spell she was under just yet.

She found the mat and got herself into an all-fours position. Having discarded her shirt and shorts at the door, she was now standing in her underwear, which was soon also discarded on the floor. Naked, her body gleamed in the ambient light. She asked me if it was okay that she was nude, I smiled and nodded, affirming she could be whatever she needed to be. Moving closer to her, I listened to her baby's heartbeat with the doppler, assuring them the baby was doing well. Placing my hand on her back, I gently touched the rhombus of Michaelis that had begun to appear there.

Just before she went into another contraction, we briefly talked about the stage she was in. With this one she let out a deep moan. To my trained ear, the sound seemed guttural, with a sense of pressure behind it. Ellie was now shaking and began questioning the process. I could see the fear creeping in, I could see her confidence begin the slippery slide, she lowered herself to the floor, rolled onto her side and covered her face with her hands. She said she wasn't coping, could I fix it, could I do something. I crawled on my hands and knees to where she lay and placed my hands on her shoulder blades from behind her, soothed her and gave her the space to collect herself. We often call this the crisis of confidence, and it is understood to likely be the transitional phase of labour. I didn't need to fix it or take it away and within seconds the next contraction hit and in one movement she returned to her all-fours position. In the next break between the contractions, that were now coming every minute or so, she stood with our help and began to furiously walk around the room. Women often resemble caged tigers at this stage, pacing back and forth, panting. They require space, both physically and mentally, to move and to open up. Drew attempted to get close, she swiped at him, pushed him away, grunted she didn't want him to touch her now. He recoiled but stayed close. He even stepped off the floor mat he stood on realising that it was her space, for a little more distance.

We watched and we waited, she continued to pace to room. I heard a soft knock at the door. I sighed deeply, of course, the team of doctors on shift would want to know what was going on. Moving quickly before they knocked again – I stepped behind the curtain and opened the door – there stood three scrubbed doctors, waiting to be invited in. I closed the door quietly behind me and positioned myself in front of it, guarding the sacred birthing space for Ellie.

I quickly briefed them on Ellie's labour status – which was all reassuringly normal, with the baby's heart rate and her vitals in good order. They questioned why Ellie was not on a CTG monitor. I calmly explained that based on my assessment, there was no indication for continuous monitoring. I was diligently using the doppler and would escalate to monitoring if I felt it was necessary. Recalling her previous birth was induced and her haemorrhage was from an extended episiotomy, I explained this labour was spontaneous with no deviations from normal at this point. I assured them I would call for support if needed. With a nod of approval, the doctors left and I felt a warm surge of empowerment run through me.

When I returned to the room, Ellie was standing by the bed, which I had deliberately positioned away from its usual spot, offering more support than a typical lying position. Aware of her past trauma associated with that bed, I aimed to make it unrecognizable from previous experiences, I adjusted its height to allowed her to rest her arms comfortably as she swayed through contractions. Now contracting every minute, she vocalised and groaned with each wave of pain. Her physical stance had altered, the baby had visibly descended, and she keenly felt the pressure of impending birth. Feeling the urge to break her waters, Ellie turned to me, desperation in her eyes. Despite my suggestion to utilise the contractions to rupture the membranes naturally, and after attempting this for two contractions, she grew increasingly frustrated. With a determined look, she insisted that I break the waters. It's challenging to reason with a woman in such as state; she was acutely aware that her baby was ready to emerge. I suggested we confirm her readiness but didn't want to lie her down. Instead, I assured her I would perform the procedure while she remained standing.

Ellie's intuition proved correct; the baby was indeed ready to make her entrance. I could feel the distinct roundness of the baby's head and the tautness of the amniotic sac, poised like a balloon waiting to pop. Encouraging Ellie to use her contractions and the pressure she felt, I gently traced my finger across the tight membrane as she exerted pressure. With her efforts, the sac ruptured, and the baby's head descended with the remainder of the contractions. Ellie now adopting a running man pose, pushed onward, her determination and strength phenomenal. Gradually the baby's head emerged with furrowed brows giving way to tightly closed swollen eyes. As the infant continued her descent, I kept one hand on the crown of the baby's head as I reached for the buzzer to call for a second midwife, to ensure adequate support for the birth. As the cheeks and chin became visible, I remained focused on Ellie's perineum, watching and protecting it with a compress. At this pivotal moment, Drew kneeled at my side, a steady presence in the room. He kept one had on Ellie's lower back, a touch she recalls later in the evening as grounding and reassuring. With the baby's head now fully emerged, I withdrew my hands and guided Drew's to prepare for the imminent catch. The second midwife tiptoed her way into the darkened room and sat quietly to the left of us, knowing not to disturb the safe space. Sensing the profound significance of the moment, I offered Ellie the opportunity to touch her baby as she made her grand entrance. Without a word, Ellie reached down, cupping her newly birthed daughter's head in her hands before gently retracting her hands back to be bed rail, a silent acknowledgement of the miracle unfolding before her.

'She is coming now,' Ellie whispered as the final contraction gripped her. With determined effort, Ellie birthed her baby into the waiting hands of her husband. Cradled in his strong, masculine grasp, the baby let out her first cry, marking her arrival earthside. In the room, the second midwife who has remained silently observing, captured the tender moment with a series of photographs depicting Drew holding his newborn daughter seconds after her birth.

This birth was untouched by intervention, free from drugs or episiotomies, devoid of perineal tears or excessive blood loss. Ellie brought her baby into the world naturally, empowered by her own strength and supported by a team that honoured her choices and respected her autonomy. In this space of trust and care, Ellie charted her own course through childbirth, embracing the journey in her own time and on her own terms.

The medical team on staff that night was shocked that she didn't need intervention. Later that evening, one of the junior doctors approached me, asking how I managed it.

'I didn't do it; she did. I just trusted that she could,' was my response to the inquisitive junior doctor. In that moment, I realised I had played a role in saving a mother from enduring more years of birth trauma. Ellie later shared with me that this birth had been a healing experience for her, a process of being put back together.

However, healing for me, as the witness to the trauma she had previously endured and that of so many others, would take much longer. Each birth leaves its mark, and the collective weight of those experiences can be overwhelming. While I was grateful to have been a part of a transformative birth for Ellie, the toll it took on me and the memories of previous traumas lingered, reminding me of the ongoing journey towards healing.

With over 2 decades of experience as a midwife, I have had the privilege of working in various maternity systems across Australia. From private to public hospitals, birth centres and maternity group practice, Aboriginal and Torres Strait Islander community health, teaching in the Bachelor of Midwifery program, and private midwifery practice including homebirth, I have witnessed the diverse spectrum of childbirth experiences. I've been a part of hundreds of beautiful and serene births, but unfortunately, I've also encountered far too many traumatic ones that have shaken me to my core.

There were numerous instances when the challenges seemed insurmountable, and the toll on my emotional wellbeing made me consider walking away more than once. The system often felt unsupportive of women and their choices, driven more by protocols and policies than true woman-centred or midwifery-centred care. Witnessing trauma suffered by women and babies on a daily basis is disheartening. However, it is the births that make a positive impact, the ones where women express gratitude for the support, advocacy and care that keep me committed to being a midwife.

I continue to do this work for the women, striving to restore their faith in their bodies, advocating for their choices and helping them find a voice. Every woman deserves a midwife who stands by her side. Despite challenges and the resistance to change within the system, I have chosen to be the voice for women, even if it comes at a personal cost. The system may persist in its ways, but I carry the burden of that struggle. Healing will take time, but the belief in the meaningful impact I've had on individual women keeps me going. I am fuelled by the hope for positive change in the future.

Growth occurs when you begin doing the things you believe you are not qualified to do.

Chapter 13

Just Brave Enough for the Next Step, Not the Whole Staircase

In the peak of the pandemic, between September and December 2022, within the midwifery team I was a part of, families endured the devastating loss or were left to cope with the severe injuries their babies sustained during childbirth. The narratives are being shared not only because they hold deep significance; they also highlight the exceptional care provided by the midwifery team I had the privilege to collaborate with. The appreciation I harbour for this committed team knows no bounds. Throughout this trying period, they extended unwavering support to one another and to the women under their care in the most exemplary manner. The resilience demonstrated by these midwives during this time is truly remarkable.

As a midwife with over 20 years of experience, I have encountered numerous births and supported countless women and their partners during their pregnancies, labours, births and postpartum journeys.

Midwife Crisis

However, these four women and the midwives that cared for them hold a special place in my story. The circumstances that led to the loss or injuries of their babies remains unknown, and despite my years in the field, there has been no medical evidence to draw conclusions about the tragedies that befell these families.

We were a team of seven midwives, supporting the families in our caseloads, and importantly, supporting each other through the daily routine and challenges we faced. The global pandemic was raging, leaving us to navigate lockdowns and spend as little time in the hospital as possible. The communication between us often occurred over the phone or through text messages. It was rare we actually saw each other face to face, having to adapt to the uncertainty of each day during these unprecedented times. We ensured that we stayed abreast of each other's caseloads and each other's wellbeing. Ad hoc meetings in the hospital cafeteria became crucial, allowing us to shed light on concerns regarding workload and allowing us to collaboratively find solutions. The cafeteria, shared by patients and staff alike was a diverse scene of hospital life; from the sick dragging IV drip poles and the elderly being wheeled in wheelchairs to doctors in scrubs and fresh new parents with tiny newborns in plastic cots.

The surgical masks we wore concealed our faces, and the many emotions we hid. Once discarded across the tables to sip at our coffee, a sense of familiarity was revealed. The masks, worn for so long now, made it easy to forget the intricate features of those we worked with so closely. Taking off the masks became a small yet significant act, allowing us to see each other's faces and the smiles we missed so much.

My midwife buddy Ruby and I, had formed a habit of having coffee together every day that we were on duty. It was a daily ritual we both looked forward to, often marked by simultaneous coffee emoji texts. The click of my heels and the squeak of her sneakers echoed through the hallway as we headed to our usual table near the window. The plan that day was to meet up with the other midwives on the team, but as on-call midwives, most of the team had been working around the clock with a very challenging and devasting outcome. Consequently, our team meeting was reduced to Ruby, Zoe and me.

Zoe arrived with palpable weariness, her complexion pale and fatigued. As she sat down, the collective heaviness that the team had been carrying for the past few weeks seemed to weigh on her even more. The nature of the Covid restrictions, coupled with increasing furlough numbers leading to short-staffed shifts, had left us feeling like we were the last ones standing amid this relentless storm. As Zoe began to open up, tears streamed down her face, mingling with a sip from her steaming almond latte.

'I'm not sure I can do this anymore,' she uttered, a vulnerability I had not seen before in her. Ruby and I understood the sentiment all too well, nodding in solidarity. I reached across the table to hold her free hand, while Ruby offered a starchy paper napkin to wipe away her tears.

'It's been a terrible week, we know. What can we do to help?' Ruby asked gently and in her best mothering voice. We recognised the upcoming day would be challenging for Zoe and the rest of the team. In that moment, our goal was to offer support, giving her time and space to express her emotions and vulnerabilities. The strength of the team lay in our unity, ready to navigate through the difficulties together.

Zoe and her team of two other midwives had recently experienced a full-term stillbirth in their caseload. It was unexpected and the parents, a young couple, had presented the day before due to decreased fetal movements. Supporting a couple so young through this devasting loss added such a profound layer of complexity to their role as midwives.

Midwife Crisis

The parents and the baby were still in the hospital and Zoe was assigned to care for them. Her responsibilities included supporting the parents in bathing and dressing their baby, as well as handling paperwork and preparing their discharge plan. It was an emotionally heavy load to carry alone. Zoe's two other teammates, who had been at the birth, had gone home to rest and recover. There was uncertainty about whether either of them would return the next day, leaving Zoe to feel the weight of the work fall on her shoulders. We came up with a plan to execute to ensure that Zoe could navigate through the tasks she needed to accomplish that day, providing her with support and assistance to carry out the responsibilities.

Midwives are primarily trained to welcome life into the world, equipped with thorough emergency procedures to prevent and to preserve life. However, when faced with the profound grief of a baby's death, there is a whole aspect of learning and understanding that formal training often overlooks. The art of sitting with grief, working within it and supporting a woman and her partner through one of the darkest days of their lives is a skill that only experience can truly teach. It isn't a comfortable skill to acquire, believe me, but it becomes an essential element of the job. More often than not, caregivers receive inadequate support. These are the individuals who are present during critical moments, tasked with finding the right words, offering comfort and facing the grieving families. They carry the weight of these experiences home with them every day. Creating a safe space for midwives to openly discuss the emotional impact of what they see, hear and go through is crucial. This space should be non-judgemental, and free from blame or shame, recognising that no-one is at fault.

Acknowledging and addressing the emotional wellbeing of healthcare professionals is essential for fostering resilience and maintaining a compassionate and supportive environment. There is a pressing need for a compassionate approach to caring for the caregivers, and unfortunately, many hospitals lack the capacity or insight to adequately support their staff. There's a notable lack of support during these catastrophic events, with referrals often leading to general counselling services not tailored to healthcare workers' specific needs. While there are hospital teams like the bereavement team dedicated to supporting grieving parents, there is limited capacity to address the emotional burden carried by the caseload midwife. As a midwife, you continuously navigate the turmoil of grief, remaining steadfastly present for others during their times of need. This grief may stem from experiencing the loss of a baby, a traumatic birth, or the challenges of the postpartum period, and also as you support families through the profound journey of new parenthood. Holding on to your own grief becomes a silent sacrifice allowing you to show up each day for someone else.

The hospital cafeteria served as our makeshift counselling office. Operating as caseload midwives, we lacked a dedicated space within the hospital, leaving us without a safe haven to retreat to. Our workspace consisted of two shared computers in the main reception area of the birth suite, accessible to 19 midwives and any other staff choosing to use that area. On numerous occasions I encountered wardsmen or cleaners using these computers during the night, browsing the internet for fast cars or puppy dogs for sale. Privacy and solitude were scarce.

The space we 'occupied' was also the main throughfare of the birth suite, making it challenging to find a private space during a moment of crisis. It often felt as though our needs were overlooked. The cafeteria become our refuge, where we sat and talked, solving midwifery challenges or simply sitting in silent solidarity. Recognising the need for a safe space, we provided support for each other, just as we did for the women in our care every day. Many times, we found solace in shared conversations and tears, especially when reflecting on the heartbreak and torment that went with unexplained or unexpected outcomes we encountered.

On that day, Ruby, Zoe and I, fully aware of the recent loss suffered by a couple, observed the intricate dance of the unwell, the sick, the elderly, those battling cancer and the medical professionals in their scrubs moving about the cafeteria unaware of the tragic events that had unfolded in the birth suite the day before. The profound impact of such moments becomes exceptionally poignant when your role is to bring life into the world. It inflicts a deep and heavy hurt, leaving a myriad of unanswered questions.

~

Covid-19 had hit Melbourne with full force, and we found ourselves in the midst of stage three lockdowns. Mask mandates, curfews and visitor restrictions were in place across all hospitals. Everyone was feeling the strain of exhaustion, with over half our workforce on furlough and those of us who remained, bore the weight of the increased workload and the heightened anxiety of each day.

We consistently donned full PPE for labour and birth, enduring the discomfort day in and day out. N95 masks, worn for an average of 12 hours a day became a constant source of physical strain, leaving marks on our faces, indentations on our noses and constantly causing our eyes to water due to the materials and chemicals used to make them. Our gowns were constructed from plastic, covering us from neck to feet, and our shoes shielded by surgical covers. Alongside the mandatory N95 masks, we also had to don protective goggles and face shields.

This ensemble induced profuse sweating, was uncomfortable and restrictive and the PPE often led to tense interactions with specialised supervisors, if not worn or removed correctly. Our hands were scrubbed and doused with sanitizing alcohol to such an extent that the cracks ran deep, causing pain, even when exposed to water.

Leaving a birth room required the meticulous process of doffing and donning PPE, an intricate routine emphasised in hospital-made videos that we were expected to watch regularly. In an effort to avoid this cumbersome process, some chose not to leave the birth room they were assigned to. Forgoing water intake, this strategy aimed to eliminate the need for bathroom breaks, and we learned to consume meals well in advance of a shift to stave off hunger.

Mandatory Covid vaccination for all healthcare workers in Australia was implemented, necessitating three doses within a specific timeframe. Not identifying as an anti-vaxxer, I initially harboured scepticism about the vaccine, particularly in the early stages of the pandemic. Concerns, especially regarding pregnant women, fuelled my apprehension. Ultimately, I chose to receive all vaccinations. Expressing my feelings was challenging at times as I sensed a lack of comprehensive, unbiased information to share with the women in our care. We were given a policy outlining the specific messaging the system wanted us to convey and upper management offered no alternative information. When women questioned it, the solution was to suggest they do their own research. Unfortunately, many didn't, instead accepting the health department's advice, receiving vaccinations through pregnancy without questioning the possible side effects.

During this period of heightened anxiety amongst the patients, there were numerous women under my care who sought reassurance about safety of the vaccines. The question lingered: was it truly safe? Personally, I grappled with uncertainty, unaware of the potential impact on their unborn babies. My responses were guided by the hospital's directives and the evidence they mandated us to provide. Each time I addressed their concerns, attempting to alleviate fears, my own overwhelming anxieties loomed. The available evidence was limited, leaving me feeling like a follower in a herd, despite my reluctance to conform, and I battled the internal conflict I had on a daily basis during this time

To this day, I remain Covid-free, never having tested positive or experiencing the illness. It seems I might be one of those rare 'unicorns' they mention. Despite providing care to women who tested positive before and during labour, being exposed to their bodily fluids, literally catching their babies, and handling blood and body parts, including spilled or squirted breastmilk, I have miraculously avoided succumbing to the virus.

Enduring the pandemic and the persistent lockdowns, felt like an unending and unyielding challenge. Our spirits were drained, stripping away the essence of genuine care. Rules underwent constant change, shifting daily and making it difficult to stay abreast of the instability of the fluctuations. Our routines were marked by daily PCR tests, alterations in PPE and constant modifications in policies attempting to keep up with the changes handed down by the government health regulators. Early in the wave of hysteria of the virus, a disheartening policy emerged, which prohibited us allowing women to use water, either bath or shower, pre or post birth due to a concern that our PPE would get wet while supervising. The inhumanity of such a restriction was profound and understandably was not followed by many midwives and eventually the entire policy was disregarded.

Amid prolonged lockdowns and heightened anxiety, it became evident that some of my colleagues chose not to get vaccinated. With the vaccination deadline approaching, midwives began to disappear from the team. One remarkable midwife I met at another establishment, with whom I collaborated on various aspects of our careers, faced significant health issues and prioritised her wellbeing. She did not outright refuse the vaccines but requested more time to decide, to research the potential effects on her already compromised immune system. After years of battling various illnesses, weight loss and infertility, she wanted to prepare herself. Unfortunately, the hospital she worked for did not permit time extensions or vaccine exemptions. When the deadline arrived, she was removed from the roster and, like many others, was no longer seen at her place of work.

It didn't occur to me at the time what had happened to those that had disappeared from our rosters. I didn't comprehend their situations or their adversity to the vaccines. It was only after spending time and discussing her case that it dawned on me that she, along with many others like her, had been forced to leave, rounded up and caged, the unvaccinated, the outcasts. Like the others, her caseload was taken over by the remaining midwives, which added to the burden of their already increased workloads and expectations.

In the writing of this book, I asked her to share her experience, which offered insight into her life and how she coped during this time. She had pleaded with management, arguing that the vaccines were detrimental to her health. She attempted to secure documents indicating her risk factors, past reactions to vaccines, and her compromised immune system, requesting an extension to ensure she was well enough to cope with the vaccines, but her efforts were ignored.

She began to realise it was difficult for others to understand her viewpoint in relation to the vaccines. She kept her opinions to herself, knowing her teammates would not understand her stance, aware that working in this field would come with judgement and a limited perspective. Before her disciplinary leave, knowing her time was running out, she kept to herself, did her work, cared for the women under her care, and limited her time at the hospital. She did not associate with anyone outside of work and spent her days off at home under strict lockdown rules.

She attempted to communicate with the management and HR departments, receiving minimal response which became less and less as the deadline loomed. Late one afternoon she was eventually contacted by her manager and was told that she could no longer attend to her patients under her care. She was not allowed on site and that she should divert her work phone to another midwife on her team. There was no discussion around the action, only that she should inform the appropriate department when she was fully vaccinated, as only then could she could return to work. Soon after this she was officially notified that she was on disciplinary leave and was instructed not to return to work until she complied with the vaccination mandate. She was informed she must comply with the mandate if she wished to retain her employment. She struggled to understand this mandate, feeling it was discriminatory and a breach of human rights and privacy. Ironically, as healthcare providers, our job is to advocate for choice and informed decision-making. She extensively reviewed Work Health & Safety policies and workplace responsibilities. Her research revealed that she would normally be entitled to an individual risk assessment, but these responsibilities seemed to be disregarded during the pandemic, and she was never allowed to undergo such an assessment related to her circumstances.

Desperate for support, understanding and connection with others who faced similar situations, she reached out to online groups filled with healthcare workers who were also unvaccinated and had recently been dismissed from their jobs. She soon found herself speaking with many others, including psychologists, physiotherapists, midwives, and nurses – all in the same position, all threatened with disciplinary action or termination unless they complied with the vaccination policy.

Each person carried their own unique and often heartbreaking story. Some had suffered significant reactions to their first Covid shot but were being pressured to receive three doses to keep their jobs. Others like herself were unable to financially survive without work. Some had sought government support for the first time in their lives, others relying on family and friends for basic amenities, they could no longer afford to buy. They were made to feel like rebellious outcasts, even though they were all dedicated healthcare workers, willing to work and desperate to return to their jobs.

Soon, one by one, the people she was communicating with began receiving emails about individual meetings with HR departments, eventually all receiving termination notices.

She received a meeting request for a Zoom call scheduled several weeks into her leave. During this meeting, she was given a chance to discuss her reasons and health concerns. She reiterated that she had not refused vaccination but had requested more time and at least the opportunity to seek advice from her specialist. After this meeting, she heard nothing for several more weeks, and her emails and phone calls remained unanswered.

By this time, the lockdown in Melbourne had forced businesses to close, with no end in sight. Her partner's small business was affected, and they were financially distressed with no income. They had gone from a double-income family to nothing. They relied heavily on family and friends, utilised savings to pay utility bills, and put food on the table for their small family. Like many others during that time, neither of them qualified for Covid hardship payments. Their relationship became strained and stressful. They resorted to buying only essential items and accepting meals made by friends. Feelings of resentment intensified, as her partner had been vaccinated but could not work, while she was forgoing the opportunity to earn income as an essential worker. She had the freedom that essential workers had, albeit minus the choice to be vaccinated. After nights of going hungry due to not having enough food for herself, opting to feed their children, she began to seriously question her decision. She felt she had no choice but to be vaccinated. It was a difficult but essential means of survival by this point, as there were no alternative employment opportunities available without vaccination status.

It took her days to come to terms with the decision. Making that phone call to the HR department was agonising and filled her with remorse. She knew it was the only way to save her relationship, her children and her career. She needed to prove a booked vaccination appointment, which she didn't have at the time of the call, so she had to arrange one at the local community centre. The next available appointment was a week away. After booking it, she called the HR department again with proof of the appointment. It was reiterated that she would need to provide evidence once the vaccination had been received. She sensed a lack of trust, that she would somehow cheat the system, she felt very patronised and beaten down, like she had surrendered to the hand that forced her. Her demeanour changed; she no longer felt connected to the job she had deeply cared for. She found it hard to find anything that made her happy or even smile during this, her bright, carefree self was gone. She began to suspect that she was just another number on the conveyor belt, which at times felt impossible to get off. She was assured that once she received the first vaccine, she could return to work. Like everyone else, she was naive enough to believe this. Later, she wished she had received that assurance in writing.

After informing the HR team that she had received the first vaccine according to the schedule, she hoped to return to work despite experiencing some severe side effects. Several days passed without any communication from them, during which she allowed herself to recover. Nine days after receiving the first dose, she received an email stating that she could not return to work until she had completed the full vaccination schedule. This news left her confused and disheartened, as it meant she had to anxiously wait for months to complete the schedule. In the meantime, she endured recurring doctor's visits, swollen lymph nodes, unexplained breast lumps, daily fevers, severe cramping and vomiting. These symptoms seemed to be a cascade of reactions that consequently appeared soon after the vaccine. To this day her armpits remain reddened and swollen, making it difficult to wear a bra on occasion or even use a roll on deodorant due to the pain. She claims that the swelling was not present prior to receiving the vaccine.

Despite her apprehensions about the second and third vaccines and the severity of her reactions, for the sake of her family, she had no choice but to proceed with booking these appointments. Her third and final vaccine was scheduled three months later. Once again, she notified the HR team and endured another prolonged wait for a response, preparing herself to return to work. A phone call from a manager came at the last minute, delivering the devastating news that she could not return to her caseload midwifery role until she provided certification of her third dose. She was accused of being disruptive and unfair to other team members, that her choices had affected everyone else. Feeling very isolated and alone, fearful of where she would be without her job, without any contact with her teammates and unsure if any of what she was told was true, she pleaded with the manager to keep her role open, assuring them that she was prepared to receive the third vaccine. In a swift turn of events, the manager's tune changed, offering her the opportunity to return to work only if she took up some shortfall shifts on a postnatal ward. The offer didn't sit well with her and she questioned the integrity of the manager's offer. How could she work on the postnatal ward with new mothers and babies, yet not return to her caseload position?

Given the financial pressure she was under, she reluctantly chose to comply with these shifts. She continued to seek answers and ultimately expressed her desire to find employment elsewhere if she could not return to her contracted role. It became evident that the hospital was critically understaffed. Despite contacting and discussing her situation with the union, she was informed that it was legal for her employer to deploy staff to other areas as needed. However, it seemed that no other caseload midwives had been 're-deployed' to work in other areas. Frustrated and depleted by the fight, she was still not brave enough to throw it all in. She needed the job and the financial stability it provided.

During her time on the ward, ironically, she contracted Covid for the first time, only two weeks after her second vaccine dose. As her symptoms worsened, she was hospitalised and transferred to another major metropolitan hospital's Covid ward, where she received oxygen support and respiratory medications. As she regained her strength and was discharged home several days later to recuperate, she constantly feared her employer would not believe her, as she now required more time off for sick leave. Ironically, being granted sick leave was not an issue. The medical certificate she submitted confirmed that she had contracted Covid and had been hospitalised for medical attention.

Midwife Crisis

Still recovering from her ordeal in the hospital, she received a call from the HR department that once again made her question the ethics of her employer. What she thought would be their first display of empathy for her health, turned into questions about which shifts she would be picking up on the postnatal ward and when. Bewildered by their insensitivity, she found it illogical. Once again, she was informed that she could not resume her duties as a caseload midwife until she had received the third vaccination. It felt like another stab in the back, twisting it a bit harder and deeper, reminding her she was still an outcast. What was perplexing and made no sense was that other midwives in their assigned roles were allowed to continue working while awaiting their final vaccine dose.

Prior to the date of her third dose, she received a statutory declaration from her GP, stating that two vaccines were sufficient and constituted full vaccination and it was strongly advised that she did not receive a third dose due to her recent reactions and weakened immune system. Hoping that this official document would satisfy her employers and enable her to delay the third vaccine, she bravely broached the subject of returning to work sooner than expected. However, her health warning was dismissed, and she was simply advised to try another brand of vaccine. She was also warned that her job remained at risk if she did not comply with the policy. Her stress intensified, manifesting in physical symptoms such as unexplained hair loss, heavy menstrual bleeding and dramatic weight loss. Mentally and physically strained, she began to question if she was fit for the demanding work of caseload midwifery. However, financial pressures fuelled her determination to provide for her family and reclaim the job she knew she was entitled to and had fought so hard to keep.

Focused on her recovery both mentally and physically, she ate nutritious meals and used her savings for Chinese and alternative therapy. Following advice, she dramatically increased her water intake and exposed herself to sunlight as often as possible. The time spent at home with her family, focusing on herself and them, is something she will forever cherish. She tells me that without her incredible partner and sister encouraging and nursing her back to health over those months, supporting her through countless appointments, and even helping her with daily tasks, she feels she might not have survived the gruelling symptoms she experienced.

Ultimately facing financial turmoil after depleting their savings on her recovery, and with the date of her third vaccine looming, she reluctantly decided to undergo the final vaccine to comply with her employer's request. Fortunately, this vaccine did not affect her immune system as severely as the first two, nor did it cause significant symptoms. Her recovery from this vaccine was less exhausting, allowing her to manage daily tasks and prepare to return to work.

Fully recovered, re-energised, and eager to return to work, she informed her colleagues of her return and, with trepidation, began to reclaim her caseload role. Despite providing the third vaccine certificate as requested, there was no response from the HR team or her manager. Her return was met with silence, and her manager continued to ignore her presence. This lack of acknowledgment underscored the impersonal nature of the workplace, making her often question if she had made the right decision to fight for a job where she felt so undervalued. What kept her driven, and still does, are the relationships and care she has for women and families. Many midwives struggle with this issue, as our role feels increasingly redundant, perceived as merely showing up and doing the job while our care settings become ever more institutionalised, marginalised and mechanical.

Below are some stories that this midwife shared with me, highlighting the heartbreak and exceptional experiences of families she cared for throughout the pandemic. The trauma endured by these women and their families during pregnancy, labour and birth is significant and warrants inclusion in this book. Midwives have been integral parts of these challenging journeys, sharing in the emotional weight of the outcomes. These stories shed light on the profound impact of the pandemic on maternity care and emphasise the importance of acknowledging and addressing the traumas faced by those navigating the complexities of childbirth during such unprecedented times.

~

Shortly after resuming her caseload position, all her interactions with pregnant women were closely examined by senior staff to ensure she was promoting certain vaccinations during pregnancy. She was frequently questioned about the information she provided during antenatal clinic appointments and felt particularly scrutinised if any of her clients declined the vaccines.

As the virus spread among pregnant women, information about the vaccines was vague and uniformly presented, directing us as medical professionals on how to communicate it. The message was clear: there were no concerns about the vaccines' safety or efficacy, and they could be administered at any stage of pregnancy. We were consistently confronted with fear-mongering about the severe consequences of not receiving at least three vaccines during pregnancy. Holding on to immense guilt about complying with this advice to keep her job, her fear and anxiety had reached such heights that she was conflicted about her understanding of the profession. The core ethos of being a midwife is to support and encourage women to make informed decisions for themselves and their babies. Yet, she felt these values slipping away as she gave advice, she had little confidence in. It became rote and mechanical, preventing her from sharing what she knew firsthand.

The early stages of the pandemic were difficult to navigate, with frequent lockdowns, regularly changing protocols, and families managing fear and uncertainty. Strict visiting rules were applied to antenatal clinics, birth suites, postnatal wards, SCNs, and NICUs across the country's maternity units, completely disrupting family-centred care. She encountered two families who had seemingly low-risk pregnancies and no history of abnormalities. Both women had received the mandated vaccines during their pregnancies and had contracted the virus in either their second or third trimesters. Sadly, both of their babies became unwell shortly after birth and were admitted to the hospital's Special Care Nursery (SCN). Ultimately, both were diagnosed with rare genetic disorders several months later.

~

A young couple she had cared for were expecting their first baby and were diagnosed with late-onset fetal growth restriction in the third trimester, often due to placental insufficiency. A planned induction allowed them to welcome their seemingly healthy baby quickly and without trauma. However, soon after birth, the baby was admitted to the SCN for being low birth weight, having low tone, being unable to feed effectively, and experiencing regular oxygen desaturations. Their baby stayed in the SCN for many weeks, growing but gaining minimal weight. Her tone remained low, and she was eventually discharged home with no clear reason for her condition.

Spending time in an SCN ward is a terrifying and exhausting experience for any parent. Holding deep gratitude for the staff who work in this field, the environment is generally busy, understaffed, and feels impersonal. As a midwife, walking into this space after having gotten to know a family for so many months prior carries a deep feeling of helplessness, especially when required to wear PPE and see only one parent at a time.

While midwifery is an ever-challenging job with unexpected outcomes, we rarely anticipate ending up in this environment when working with ideally low-risk families. We do our best to support clients during this time, but there is a sadness carried for the unknowns ahead when there is a sick baby involved. There are no excited siblings or family members to meet, no privacy to support breastfeeding or bonding, no laughter over shared cups of tea. Just deafening silences among the alarming machines and the agonising wait for their baby to get better, to take the next step towards going home with them.

While supporting another family shortly after her experiences with the first two, a woman contracted Covid during her 31st week of pregnancy, soon after receiving her final vaccine. She relied on natural health remedies and remained isolated for the recommended duration. After a normal labour and full-term birth, the baby did not respond as expected, showing poor muscle tone and requiring oxygen. Within an hour of birth, the baby was placed on CPAP (continuous positive airway pressure) and admitted to the SCN for additional breathing support. The baby remained significantly hypotonic, with low muscle tone, appearing and acting like a floppy, limp rag doll. This condition, known as 'floppy infant syndrome,' is rare. Despite many weeks and numerous tests, there was no improvement, though the test results were normal. Eventually, the baby was able to go home but continued to be tube-fed due to the risk of aspiration from bottle feeding. The future looked challenging, involving physiotherapy, feeding tubes, and wheelchairs, with the possibility that the little girl might never speak.

$\sim$

Understanding how two healthy women with no concerning family histories or previous drug or alcohol dependencies could face such challenges was difficult and heartbreaking. When they are discharged from the SCN, there is no requirement for their midwife to visit, as the babies have likely passed the age of two weeks, the standard home visit period for caseload midwives. This lack of follow-ups or closure with these women felt wrong, especially since postnatal care and home visits are essential aspects of caseload care.

As a midwife caring for a family with a baby admitted to SCN, there is always a lingering sense of dread. You question every aspect of the care you provided. Did you miss something? Could this have been prevented? What went so wrong? Will they find any answers today? How do I comfort this family? There are countless sleepless nights of worry, knowing these clients go home each day without their baby, grappling with the same questions. Suddenly, you find yourself doubting the deep, intrinsic trust you once had in the process of pregnancy and birth.

Expecting the unexpected is an inherent part of being a midwife, something for which you are never fully prepared. How a normal day can suddenly turn into the most devastating tragedy remains inexplicable.

∼

Hearing from one of her young, healthy couples in early labour always brought her immense joy. The excitement, joy and anticipation that accompany a midwife heading to meet her clients at the birth suite are unparalleled. Her colleague had met the couple at the birth suite, explained that their midwife was on her way, and began the admitting paperwork, settling them into the birth room. She arrived to take over the care of her clients.

During the process of commencing the admission CTG, her colleague was unable to locate the fetal heartbeat. Assuming there was a malfunction with the monitor or that the baby was not in the expected position, a fetal scalp electrode was placed on the baby's head. Panic and confusion filled the room as the monitor indicated non-reassuring features. Without leaving the room, the two midwives pressed the emergency buzzer to alert the birth suite team. A doctor performed a bedside ultrasound, revealing decreased heart activity and rapid decline. The CTG monitor confirmed the baby's deterioration.

An emergency ensued, and the two midwives, along with a team of doctors and specialised pediatricians, urgently prepared for a

Midwife Crisis

category 1 caesarean section. She remembers the panic and rush of adrenaline as they ran into the operating theatre, following the bed that was being pushed at full speed. There was no time to change into scrubs; apart from the two surgeons waiting in the cold, clinical operating room, all other medical personnel were in their regular clothes.

After what seemed like an eternity, the mother was given general anaesthesia, and a scalpel sliced across her tight, round abdomen. Seconds later, a perfectly still baby girl was placed in her arms. There was no heartbeat. The room fell silent, except for the hushed tones of the doctors who began conducting CPR. Each person held their breath, waiting. Assigned to document each stage of the resuscitation, she yelled for them to speak louder, unable to hear through their tightly fitted masks and the ringing in her ears. The silence was deafening. As the mother remained under general anaesthesia, unaware of what was unfolding, she stepped closer to the bed, squeezed the young woman's hand, and held back tears, wishing the baby back to life through the incredible efforts of the doctors.

Watching in disbelief, she observed the very best doctors performing CPR on the tiny lifeless body. The timer on the resuscitation cot glowed 14 minutes – they had been resuscitating the baby for a full 14 minutes. It seemed as though they didn't want to give up. Then, suddenly at 14 minutes and 4 seconds, a faint heartbeat returned. The team stabilised the baby with further resuscitation efforts, ensuring her lungs could continue to support her breathing, sending oxygen to her brain. One of the doctors, while suturing the mother's abdomen, looked up from the operating table and muttered in a hushed tone that the father needed to be updated.

Knowing it was her responsibility, she left the theatre and stood briefly in the airlock space, allowing herself to take a deep breath for the first time since she had arrived at work that day. Knowing the baby was far from stable and would be spending a considerable amount of time in the NICU, she gathered herself, wiped her sweaty palms on her pants, and moved slowly towards the waiting room. It's a tremendous effort to inform a parent that their baby has been born but is in a very unstable condition. They are immediately elated but the colour and excitement suddenly drain from their face when you mention the need for NICU. It is even more difficult to help them control their emotions when they are not allowed to see their partner or their baby due to restrictions.

Sadly, the baby remained in very poor condition due to profound acidosis and lack of oxygen during those prolonged minutes. Despite being rushed to the NICU and receiving maximum ventilator support, an adrenaline infusion, and anticonvulsant therapy, she could not be saved. The most painful part of being a midwife is sitting at the bedside of a mother waking from the haze of general anaesthesia, asking if her baby is okay. These are the moments when the world literally stops. You can see someone's heart breaking, and delivering that news is beyond any training found in a textbook.

Later that evening, the baby's endotracheal tube was removed, and she died peacefully in her mother's arms, with her father holding them both.

When it's over, it's hard to believe what you walked into that day. You are left wandering the dark hallways as night descends over the hospital, hearing faint cries of other babies being settled by their mothers. You pass through the bustling wards preparing for handover, not knowing where to go or what to do. It feels wrong to go home and leave this family in the care of strangers who did not witness the tragedy that unfolded only a few hours ago, but she also knew her presence was not needed. A chance encounter in the hallway with a pastoral care worker encouraged her to leave, asking if she needed someone to come and get her, if she was okay to drive home. She walked out of the hospital that night, alone and numb.

The reality of the situation finally began to sink in as she walked into her own house, greeted with a warm embrace by her partner and an offer to run her a bath. As she sank her tired body into the heat of the water, the numbness began to lift, and she finally had the space to sob uncontrollably in her own bathroom. Returning to work the next day and the day after, unable to stand being at home alone with her thoughts, she needed the busyness of the job to keep her mind from going to the darkest place. She was angry and heartbroken, unable to comprehend how something like this could happen to someone so healthy, without explanation. Her partner and the midwives in her team encouraged her to take time off, but she explained that she did not want to, continuing to distract herself by caring for other families. Afraid that if she wasn't there, the unthinkable would happen. She knew she wasn't to blame, yet she blamed herself and continued to search for answers.

Caring for bereaved parents is as exhausting as it is humbling, and at times it can leave you feeling utterly helpless. Visiting bereaved parents is often overwhelming. Entering their sacred space where they would have held and soothed their newborn, seeing empty feeding chairs you would have supported them in, untouched cots and prams, and unwrapped gifts and pastel-coloured flowers scattered around the living rooms – these sights can be deeply affecting. A feeling of shame often washes over you, not having any answers when they begin to question why it happened to them. She began to question everything she knew about birth, analysing everything she was saying to other prospective parents, while the fear of repercussions loomed over her. Would she be held responsible? Would she have to justify her actions? She was terrified of facing a coroner's case, knowing every piece of advice and documentation she had written for this family would be scrutinised.

It's the psychological stress that does so much damage and is not often recognised or spoken about in the midwifery profession – the waiting to be blamed for the outcome.

Soon after, she gave up teaching the antenatal classes she had so dearly loved. She was unable to bear singing the praises of the magic and wonder of birth when nothing could explain such a freak accident. She feared the inevitable question: what if something goes wrong? She wanted to scream that something did go wrong and no-one could fix it, not even her.

The couple declined a post-mortem exam, so it remains unknown how or why this baby died. There was no coroners court, no requests for explanation by her employer, no reprimand on her. She was not reported to the regulatory board.

As the weeks passed by and the days rolled on, her work continued. Preparing and caring for families meeting their babies, she often thought of the families who had lost their babies. She continued to care, support, teach and listen, learning every day what it means to care and to be cared for. The support she received from her team of colleagues and her family gave her the strength to carry on being the midwife she always had been. As caregivers, we get up and ride the waves – but sometimes we drown in them. In the hardest times, we search for a lifeguard, but there is no-one there to help us out of the rolling waves. She received no formal debriefing for what she experienced during this tragic event, and there was no checking in from management. Grieving this loss during the pandemic was exceptionally difficult. She often spent shifts alone, enduring long, gruelling hours only to go home to isolation, with family who didn't understand the depth of her grief and sadness. There were no support or comfort measures to lean on when they were needed the most.

The fleeting comments of 'make sure you look after yourself' seemed to hold little meaning when taking a day off would be unthinkable due to the burden it would place on the rest of the team. Despite these feelings, she continued to show up for work each day, braving the birth suite with labouring women, even though she was plagued with fear and constantly doubted her skills and ability to continue.

Midwife Crisis

As professionals, the essential workers, the birth keepers, we were left without care or tenderness for events that continue to leave deep scars.

~

These experiences during the height of the Covid-19 pandemic are truly heart-wrenching and showcase the challenges and complexities faced by healthcare professionals and patients alike. The stories shared with me underscore the profound impact of the pandemic on pregnancies, births and the emotional wellbeing of families and the midwives involved.

The cases she describes, particularly those involving babies with rare genetic disorders and the heartbreaking stillbirth, highlight the intricate interplay between maternal and fetal health and the raging pandemic. It's evident that the uncertainties and fear surrounding the virus added an additional layer of stress to an already sensitive and vulnerable period. This stress was felt not only by expecting families, but gravely by the midwives and doctors involved directly with the care of these families.

The difficulties we commonly encountered during this time in our careers and lives in advocating for proper care, the dismissive attitudes of senior level healthcare practitioners, and the subsequent insensitive revelation of fetal demise, underscore systemic challenges and the issues of moral injury that exists within the healthcare system.

It's clear that providing compassionate care in an environment such as these, fraught with fear and uncertainty, is incredibly challenging. The toll these experiences take on your professional and personal wellbeing can be profound, leaving lasting imprints on your emotional resilience and sense of self.

Stories such as these highlight the need for ongoing improvement in healthcare systems, communication protocols and support structures for both healthcare providers and patients. The emotional toll on healthcare professionals, as well as the need for empathy and understanding in times of crisis, is a crucial aspect that warrants attention and reform.

.

Being okay does not
always mean being alright.
It's okay to come undone, for it is
only in the darkness that you can
discover the power of your own
light.

Chapter 13 ½

Sleep, Sex, Food and the Darkness

As an on-call midwife, the routine in your life is anything but regular. However, amidst the unpredictability, there are a few constants that you can rely on for consistency – sleep, sex and food. These elements do not follow a specific order or any conventional sequence. It would have been uncommon to have spent more than two consecutive nights in your own bed in a week. Being on call means that you would be available day and night, at any given moment. Sometimes you worked until the sun rose the next day. Here is my 'recipe' of my life on call and some strategies I use for winding down and relaxing after the events of the day or night.

Sleep – often broken, many times a night. Taken whenever, and wherever, as needed. My bed was the preferred place although I have had naps in cars, on floors, lounges, upright chairs, spare birth suite beds and once even in a small tin shed on a mattress on an isolated property awaiting a baby. You adapt to surviving on minimal sleep and make the most of what you have. Eventually fatigue takes its toll and cherished days off become a respite. Mandatory sleep-ins mark the occasions and numerous meals are consumed in bed.

Midwife Crisis

Sex – is a necessity when feeling excessively tired, as it helps in inducing sleep naturally by releasing oxytocin. While having a willing partner is beneficial, solo intimacy is also satisfying. After eating and showering, take me by the hand and guide me to the bed. Engage in lovemaking until all worries fade away, allowing me to drift into the deep slumber I long for.

Food – is essential and vital when feeling excessively tired, as it aids in inducing sleep. I have always found it challenging to sleep on an empty stomach. It is common for me to call ahead to notify that I was on my way home, requesting a nutritious and fulfilling meal to be prepared upon my arrival. Whether living with a partner or solo, having meals ready or easy to prepare is a crucial requirement of being an on-call midwife. After a busy shift of supporting birth, it is understandable to feel drained. You likely haven't hydrated enough or eaten at appropriate times and at such times, making food decisions can feel overwhelming, especially when your brainpower is depleted.

Darkness – block-out curtains are a must in allowing the darkness to descend on you when your eyes grow heavy, signalling the readiness to shut down and off. Essential oils, calming sleep music or white noise can help drown out the noises of everyday life happening around you. Darkness, metaphorically, also creeps in when you realise and recognise witnessing pain, distress and trauma regularly is far from normal.

Trees lose their leaves every year,
they shed and still stand tall.
They patiently wait for the sun to
shine upon them once more.

Chapter 14

I'm Not Strong,
I Am Surviving

Surviving is a choice. Recently, my lifelong girlfriend Rachael had the words 'survive or thrive' tattooed along her forearm. She is now thriving while she survives, but the past 3 years has been a battlefield filled with landmines for her. She has endured and survived breast cancer, her mother's passing after years of the debilitating disease that is motor neurone disease, and most recently, on top of all of this, the breakdown of her 23-year marriage. We have known each other since we were 10 years old but didn't become real friends until our first year of high school. I walked up to her one day in the school yard and rescued her, so she tells me, from the nerdy group and welcomed her into the cool girl gang, probably one of the bravest things I ever did, choosing her. Together we have faced all the best and worst things that life could throw at us. She picked me up and dusted me off when my first marriage fell apart, she supported me through the tough days of finding myself again. We have supported each other through pregnancies, births, the seemingly endless toddler years and the rollercoaster ride that goes along with raising teenagers. Our friendship has additionally endured navigating the tidal waves of our careers, losing parents and grandparents and the loss of the business I had worked so hard for. She remains a constant presence, the calm that guides me through the highs and lows and everything that is in between. I believe surviving any of it wouldn't have been as manageable without each other. While she embraces a new life as a single woman, managing co-parenting with her estranged husband, navigating the challenges that comes with separation, post-cancer survival and losing a parent, I have not fared so well during this season of my life. I am merely surviving in a situation that I had control over. I made choices that steered me into oncoming traffic. At times, it felt like my head was being held underwater, but she is always there to lift me back to the surface. The friendship we have is beyond anything I could have imagined back then, when I was that sassy 13-year-old girl asking her to be my friend.

In 2021, I met Serena, who was married to Rich and mum to Zane whom she had given birth to, two years prior at the same hospital she was now attending for her second pregnancy. Her first labour and birth induced for postdates at 41 weeks had ended in a vacuum extraction due to a delay in second stage. They had just finished renovating their dream house in the inner suburbs of Melbourne when Serena sought care from my colleague for her second pregnancy and due to Covid restrictions, I initially didn't have the opportunity to get to know her well. Many of her appointments were conducted over the phone or online, causing frustration and anxiety as she felt the frequency of the in-person visits were insufficient – a mandate imposed during the pandemic. It wasn't until the later stages of her pregnancy that she started coming to the hospital for her visits and it was at 36 weeks that I finally had the chance to meet her. We immediately clicked and during our weekly appointments, we found ourselves engaging in face-to-face conversations about fashion, life and house styling.

The connection was effortless, as if we had been friends for a lifetime already. We bonded over the shared experience of having best friends who had battled breast cancer. She expressed her admiration and love for her friend who after undergoing a double mastectomy, was now expecting her first baby. Serena was thrilled at the prospect of their babies being the same age. Like most second-time mums she had more confidence in her ability to birth and was less afraid of the unknown, but still needed guidance and support. She wanted to labour spontaneously this time and wanted to allow her pregnancy to go to its full length. Despite experiencing the typical aches and pains of pregnancy, Serena managed to carry her pregnancy with grace. Her radiant skin, shiny thick blonde hair and well-rounded bump garnered significant attention. Surprisingly, her only grievance stemmed from comments suggesting that she didn't appear as if she were about to give birth any day now.

She came into labour in the early hours of the morning, calling me around 2 am with contractions and a slight amount of bleeding. She laboured at home until around 9 am, coming into the hospital once Zane had been settled with his grandma. She entered the birth suite radiating confidence, greeting everyone with a warm smile and a cheerful 'good morning'. For her truly it was a good morning – she was in labour, experiencing effective contractions and adorned in her chosen birthing dress.

Over the next few hours we worked together, she utilised her TENS machine for pain relief and embraced mobility as a crucial part of her birthing process. She moved gracefully around the room, leaning on various surfaces and relying on the support of Rich as the intensity of the contractions steadily increased. In her birthing dress, Serena exuded a remarkable blend of strength, grace and the odd profanity when a particular nasty contraction hit. She did, however, navigate the fast and furious labour with resilience and determination.

During her previous labour experience, Serena expressed feeling confined to the bed, tethered to the monitors and machines. She felt out of control and that the experience didn't belong to her. She was told what to do and when to do it. Determined to offer her a more liberating birthing experience, I encouraged her to move freely around the room, and use the shower and bathroom as she pleased. Observing her cues, I could sense a pivotal moment when she transitioned from talking and smiling to a quieter and more focused state, signalling the time of birth was nearing. As Serena approached the final stages of labour, she pleaded with me to break her waters, as they had not yet released. Sceptical of my visual assessment that I thought she was close, she requested a cervical check to confirm that she was fully dilated. After some gentle persuasion and navigating through a few more contractions that saw her take to her knees and reporting pressure, I agreed to break her waters. I released the amniotic sac that gently held her baby. The process of doing this requires delicate assistance, as some sacs are more resilient than others. Following this intervention, Serena positioned herself on the large double bed in the room, assuming an all-fours stance. With two powerful pushes, Serena welcomed her baby boy into the world on a clear sunny day.

Overwhelmed with tears and grins that seemed permanent, Serena and Rich recognised that their family was now complete. In a symbolic gesture Serena instructed Rich to dispose of the birthing dress, signifying the closure of that chapter and the beginning of a new phase in their lives.

This narrative leads me to the story of Katie, Serena's best friend. Much like my own enduring friendship with Rachael, Katie and Serena's connection began in early childhood and they faced numerous trials through life's challenges and bitter twists. At the age of 32, Katie received the life-altering diagnosis of breast cancer, compounded by a positive result for the BRCA gene. Faced with an incredibly courageous decision, she opted for a double mastectomy. Enduring chemotherapy and radiation, her body was subjected to considerable strain, with potential threats to her fertility now looming.

I'm Not Strong, I Am Surviving

Despite the adverse effects of the drugs on her reproductive capacity, Katie and her husband Jacob, swiftly decided to embark on the journey of trying for a baby. Miraculously, after just a few attempts she conceived naturally. Alone in Western Australia, they made the choice to relocate back to Melbourne, seeking the support and security of family and friends to navigate the remainder of the pregnancy. Katie's family resided in an inner suburb of Melbourne where she grew up and where her family home still stood. In the 30th week of her pregnancy Katie and Jacob undertook the challenging cross-country journey, driving in manageable blocks of 2–4 hours per day over 2 weeks. Upon reaching Melbourne, they were welcomed with overwhelming love and a joyous homecoming.

Serena had introduced Katie and I via phone and email a few weeks earlier. I was fortunate enough to have Katie under my care at the hospital, although not without its challenges. Due to her medical history, having battled breast cancer and undergone the double mastectomy, she was initially considered high risk. Advocating fiercely for her need for continuity of care, I eventually persuaded the head of obstetrics to allow her care with my caseload team.

Our first meeting took place in my small windowless clinic room amid the pandemic. Katie struck me as slender and fine boned, a naturally stunning woman. Her make-up free face, clear and tanned skin, and calming presence made everyone feel at ease with her. She appeared confident and controlled. Her long dark hair was loosely tied into a ponytail that swayed as she walked, her bright green eyes sparkled, and behind the mask, I could tell her smile would light up a room. Katie's baby bump was barely noticeable, concealed underneath her black cotton overalls. This was the beginning of our journey together to meet her much-wanted baby.

I met Jacob via FaceTime, a common occurrence during the pandemic and then we met in person very late in the pregnancy. Both were enthusiastic about an unmedicated, minimal intervention, natural birth – precisely the type I like to support. Armed with hypnobirthing techniques learned in their course, they were ready for the birthing experience they had diligently planned and envisaged.

Katie was unvaccinated, due to both a medical exemption and a choice she had chosen for herself and her baby. This choice stirred controversy at the hospital, leading to judgement, pressure and unnecessary comments from some healthcare professionals. There were even discussions suggesting she might not be able to give birth at the hospital due to her unvaccinated status, although thankfully, this never materialised. Katie, resilient and assertive, consistently defended her choices, and I supported her unwaveringly.

During Melbourne's strict lockdown rules, one of the most stringent in the world at the time, pregnant and birthing women, including Katie, faced significant challenges and restrictions to their human rights. The restrictions took a toll on many individuals, making the already complex experience of pregnancy and birth even more taxing.

Katie was healthy and her pregnancy seemed to coast along. She spent her days doing yoga, mediations and planning her birth, and she continued to work remotely for her employer in WA. She prepped her body and her baby for their journey. She kept herself safe and close to home, attempting to avoid any contact with the virus that was raging around her.

As Katie's due date neared, I assured her that it was entirely normal for first-time mothers to go past their due dates. Only 5 percent of babies are born on due dates and the average gestation is 41 weeks plus 2 days. This understanding kept her from feeling overly concerned, and we maintained regular check-ins to monitor her and the baby's wellbeing. She cooperated with necessary monitoring appointments but casually declined induction and any intervention such as stretch and membrane sweeps.

I'm Not Strong, I Am Surviving

However, as her 41st week approached, she began to feel the pressure from the system and her family, leading her to question whether she should opt for an induction. I remained a source of support, presenting her with choices and guidance. To ensure she was well informed, I provided her with hospital policies, allowing her to make informed decisions and decline induction if she chose to do so. Despite Katie's resolve, the pressure persisted, primarily from the obstetric team regularly monitoring her in the unit. She often felt like she was dodging metaphorical missiles, navigating the ongoing recommendations for induction. The obstetric team's insistence clashed with Katie's desire for a natural birth, creating a testing and tense dynamic as her pregnancy continued.

This is the point where Serena's role in the story becomes significant. It's essential to recall that Katie had undergone a double mastectomy, making it impossible for her to breastfeed her own baby. Katie and Serena had come to an agreement that Serena would provide breastmilk for this baby for the first 8 weeks of its life. Serena was still breastfeeding her own babe at the time, and she was one of those women who produced copious amounts of breastmilk. When Katie reached her 35th week of pregnancy, Serena began expressing her breastmilk and storing it. Her own baby had dropped a feed by this stage, so it was easy for Serena to continue the supply by expressing this feed at night and storing the milk. The milk was being stored lovingly in breastmilk bags, diligently labelled and dated by Serena. When she reached a certain volume, she would take the bags of frozen milk to Katie's parents' house and store it in their deep freeze.

I got to see this amazing gift one day on a postnatal visit. It truly is the meaning of friendship when you see what one woman would do for another. Hundreds and hundreds of bags of frozen milky goodness that would ensure this baby had the right start in life.

Later, I learned that the two of them would frequently engage in early morning conversations via phone calls or texts. During those moments when Serena was up expressing milk, Katie, dealing with pregnancy insomnia, would join in. In these quiet hours, they shared laughter and discussed the trials and tribulations of motherhood. Their bond was so strong that they instinctively knew when the other was awake. I was told that this connection continued to thrive during their postpartum journey, emphasising the enduring support and understanding they provided each other.

At 41 weeks and 5 days of pregnancy, Katie, overwhelmed by fear that she was putting her baby at risk, and worn down by pressure exerted by the system, found herself wrestling with the difficult decision to proceed with the induction of labour.

Coercive language in maternity systems is widespread and often used to persuade women to consent to interventions. While interventions such as inductions have their place in ensuring the safety of some mothers and babies, relying on outdated, one-size-fits-all algorithms from decades-old studies is not necessarily evidence-based. It's not limited to inductions; it extends to procedures like vaginal examinations, CTG monitoring, and fetal scalp electrodes. For example, the phrase 'it's just a little clip that attaches to your baby's head, it helps us monitor the baby better' downplays the procedure and omits potential risks or alternatives. Such language doesn't empower women to decline; it fails to inform them of the risks, like the fact that a metal screw is being attached to their baby's head.

It is not uncommon for women to experience some level of informal coercion during their pregnancy, labour or birth. This practice is deeply ingrained in the system, and little has been done to address it. In my years of practising midwifery, I have seen no significant change. In fact, it has worsened and, in my opinion, significantly contributes to the culture of birth trauma.

The discussion that unfolded between Katie, Jacob and the obstetrician seemed to imply that that their time had run out, that there was no alternative and that Katie's body was not capable of labour now.

Regrettably, the way this discussion is usually framed can be distressing for women and their partners, instilling doubt in their minds, suggesting that their bodies are not capable of carrying pregnancy to its full term and that their bodies have somewhat failed them by not initiating labour within the timeframe that is expected. Conversations like these often amplify the fear that their baby may be at an increased risk of complications or even death.

Following this distressing conversation and pressure to go ahead with an induction, Katie and Jacob agreed. The doctor and my colleague who had been there that day collaborated on initiating the induction process which was scheduled to commence the next day.

By the time they had left the hospital later that day, Katie was physically and emotionally drained and overwhelmed. She sensed that something was amiss, attributing it initially to exhaustion and stress. However, a rapid Covid test revealed that she was positive, despite having no symptoms other than feeling run-down and tired. After taking a long bath, she retreated to bed allowing herself to have a much-needed cry. Surprisingly, all other family members tested negative. This unexpected turn of events threw a significant spanner into the plans. The positive results for Covid meant that she would be required to use an isolation room in the birth suite for her labour and birth, that her induction would take place in a designated area for Covid-positive patients and that all care providers would need to be donned in full PPE. Jacob would also need to test negative to attend the hospital with her for her induction, as well as her labour and birth.

The following letter is Katie's description of her induction, her labour, the birth and the events that occurred. This letter was written by Katie to herself and her baby, which she gave me permission to incorporate into her story.

Midwife Crisis

To our baby,

Our journey together was a miracle and one that I had dreamed of, but thought would never eventuate. I was so sacred at the start to know you were there in my tummy, floating and waiting to meet us. The story I'm about to tell you is the story of the days leading up to labour and birth, which was not at all how I had dreamt it was going to be. But we made it through, and I am grateful that you guided me to a place we went together. When we moved to Melbourne and were accepted to the hospital for care, I was lucky enough to be in the, as I called it the 'special mummy's club'. We had our own midwife, and she really cared about us – you, me and Daddy. Let me first tell you just how grateful both Daddy and I were to have met and ended up in her care. She was an absolute dream to have with us on our journey as first-time parents. Every appointment, phone call, email or text, I felt supported and listened to, she empowered us with knowledge along every step of the pregnancy, birth and during those first newborn weeks. I honestly am not sure how we could have got through what we did if she wasn't there for us. Unfortunately, I can only describe your birth as an unnecessarily traumatic experience for me and your dad.

I wanted to tell you and to write down what we went through together as I know you won't really remember it. We wrote this from our perspective of what happened in the lead up and the day you were born because I truly hope the experience we had, never happens again and that no other mum and dad must be put through what we went through. I want to be able to let it go and yet I want to remember the first time I saw you, the first time I held you and the first time you laid on my chest.

Our due date was July 8th. We had planned and prepared for a 'natural' birth, and we wanted to go into labour when you were ready. Leading up to our 40th week, our midwife discussed with us options of going past the due date. We knew most babies are born after due dates, so we were okay to let you go to when you felt it was time to come. We knew some of the risks this might have but we felt safe with our choice. We agreed to try and give it until 41 weeks (which was our decision), at which point we would happily start thinking about an induction process if you were being a little stubborn. You were born in the time of the Covid-19 pandemic. It was a virus that spread throughout the world that locked people in their houses for weeks and weeks. Daddy and I came back to Melbourne just before it hit, and we were locked down in the house with Nanny and Poppy and all our family. We all were looking forward to you arriving, but sad you would be born during these silly lockdowns.

But at 10 days past your due date, I tested positive for this virus called Covid-19. I had caught the horrible infection. I wasn't too sick but I still had to take precautions to keep you and everyone else safe. I was told I needed to go into the hospital for monitoring to ensure you were okay, which I did. All the scans and monitoring I did show that you, our baby, was completely fine and happy inside me. The doctors and midwives in the Covid ward encouraged me to bring you on, to be induced. I wasn't sure I wanted this to happen, and I felt I was pushed into making this decision. Our midwife, Daddy and I all spoke about it and we decided the first thing was to check and see if you were ready. They checked my cervix first on the Wednesday that I was 41 weeks +5 days. I was very unsure about having an induction but with lots of talking and a few scary conversations with the doctors, we decided to go along with the induction to bring you on. We agreed to the balloon process, which would be the next day, when I would be 41 weeks and 6 days pregnant. I was still really scared, and I wasn't sure I wanted to go through with it. Daddy, Nanny and Poppy, all thought it was a good idea and so did the doctors at the hospital.

Daddy and I were put in the Covid ward for the balloon induction, this is where they put a tiny little balloon inside of me and blow it up to help labour begin. It was a way of forcing you out of me. The balloon went smoothly, it hurt of course, but it wasn't too bad. I was then monitored for an hour, to see if you were okay with the tiny balloon near your head, before being sent home. No-one stayed in the room with us though which I thought was strange seeing they were so concerned at your wellbeing for being so late. I was feeling so good and happy that we were going to meet you soon. But then we got the shock of our lives. Lots of doctors and midwives came in to say your heartbeat had 'dropped'. I didn't know what they meant by this. I was so scared your heart had stopped beating. Daddy was so scared he nearly fainted then and there in the chair. They told me to get back on the bed so that the balloon could be taken out. I did what I was told, and the balloon was quickly whipped out of me. I was really scared now and so confused. One of the doctors was about to put a drip in my hand when the head doctor stormed in and told everyone to stop what they were doing, she was happy with your heartbeat on the monitor. I even saw your little heartbeat on the monitor, it was perfect. This made me relax a bit, Daddy was still very white and scared. The doctor said to everyone that it wasn't necessary to take out the balloon, she was a bit angry and none of the other doctors and midwives in the room answered her — they were all very quiet. It was annoying that this had happened, but I'm secretly glad we didn't need it in the end. It wasn't a very nice experience having the balloon in the first place.

The monitor told us you were okay, you were always okay, the thingy on my tummy had slipped off and they weren't monitoring your heartbeat from the right place. That was all that happened. I will always wonder if someone had been in that room with us that day, would any of that happened? The doctors then gave me some options. We could have the balloon reinserted — I was not going through that again — or the other option was to meet you by a C-section. I was so confused, and I just didn't know what to do.

Not having our midwife rostered on that day, we were unsure. We felt we needed to talk to her, get her view on what had happened, and plan from there. We called her as soon as we had a private moment. We requested to go home, after we spoke to her, which the doctor said we could, and we agreed to come back tomorrow for further monitoring and to make a plan that suited us. We still needed time to digest this big day, talk to Nanny and Poppy and be at home. I wanted to go home to check in on you. I wanted to have a bath, rub my tummy and have you kick away as the warm water soothed us. I knew you would help me decide when we could just be us.

It was Friday morning now and both I and Daddy had a restless night. Throughout the night we discussed how we should meet you. After much deliberation, we made the tough choice to opt for the C-section. Although it was not the ideal way, I wanted to welcome you, time was running out. We returned to the Covid ward and were able to see and talk with our midwife, which helped us finalise our decision. The doctors were worried that I was now reaching 42 weeks pregnant, and not really knowing what had happened when they had put the balloon in, no-one could give us a clear explanation and that's what scared us the most. We just wanted you to be safe and here with us. I kept hearing the words from the doctors that you could be in danger staying in for so long.

A doctor that we had not met previously arrived to inform us that there were some issues preventing us from having the C-section that day, so we were rescheduled for Saturday morning at 7:30 am. Despite feeling very nervous and a little bit unsure that I had made the right decision, I was worried now, waiting another day after all that had happened. They kept telling me the risk of waiting this long.

It was Friday night around 6 pm when I began to feel the first signs of you choosing your birth date. You were ready, and I went into labour – how I had always expected it to happen. The contractions started mildly, and around 10 pm they had increased at which point I called our midwife, and we decided it was time to head to the hospital. Daddy and I were so excited, marvelling at the fact that you had chosen this moment – perhaps sensing something we couldn't. We diligently practised all the hypnobirthing techniques we had learned, preparing ourselves for the journey ahead. At the hospital we were greeted by our midwife, I was so glad she was there, she was going to take care of us. The labour was intense with contractions becoming increasingly difficult to manage. Daddy was by my side, providing massages, assisting me in moving and helping me in and out of the shower.

We found ourselves in an isolation room, where we were not permitted to leave. Our midwife was adorned in full Covid protection gear, resembling a scientist from a movie. A special walkie talkie was provided in the room for us to call for assistance if needed, but our midwife remained in the room with us throughout, offering continuous support and encouragement. After what felt like an eternity in labour, I asked to be checked and informed me that I was 2 cm dilated. I was so disappointed, I really thought I was almost ready to have you. Knowing it would be many more hours to go, we remained hopeful and decided to let things progress naturally through the night.

By around 3 am, exhaustion set in and I found myself in tears seeking help from Daddy and our midwife, who helped us get into comfortable positions

Midwife Crisis

and offered lots of support. Despite all our efforts I was still 2 cm when I was re-examined. We were all confused as to why progress had stalled, especially considering the intensity of the contractions, which were further complicated by your persistent kicks to my ribs. After attempting various methods of pain relief such as the gas, the TENS machine and some horrible water injections, the pain became unbearable. I reached a point where I simply couldn't cope any longer and Daddy was equally distressed seeing me in such agony.

Feeling utterly worn out and exhausted, and with our scheduled C-section looming just a few hours away, I mustered up the courage to ask if we could proceed with the surgery immediately. Recognising my distress and understanding the extent of my pain, our midwife helped us by talking about having some other pain relief. We discussed the option of having an epidural so I could rest prior to the surgery. She provided us with all information about epidurals including their potential effects on you.

When a doctor entered the room, one that we had not seen before, I was relieved that there was some hope of help and relief from the pain. She appeared kind and genuinely concerned for us. She seemed to understand the pain I was in and despite the intense contractions I was experiencing, she asked me why I wanted to have surgery. I had to explain my reasons, I had to justify for wanting to go ahead with the C-section now. She agreed with me and assured me that she would notify the other doctors and the rest of the team to prepare the theatre. Unfortunately, after she left the room, we never saw her or anyone from the surgical team again until much later.

There was no immediate action from our conversation with the doctor and no response to our persistent requests for follow up via the walkie talkie phone, nobody arrived to prepare me for the surgery we were promised. I was left to endure the distressing labour for another 2 hours. At this point, desperate for relief, we requested an epidural. Our midwife continued to communicate our urgent need for pain relief through the walkie talkie to the other staff, but the epidural never arrived. Throughout this ordeal she worked tirelessly to keep me calm while attending to Daddy who was exhausted, hungry and upset to see me in this pain. Together we shed many tears in the face of this overwhelming situation.

I'm Not Strong, I Am Surviving

Our midwife had to advocate fiercely for every single request that night, and I couldn't comprehend why this was necessary. I was left wondering why I had to endure unnecessary distress for so long, and why our pleas went unanswered. Out of frustration and almost reaching breaking point attempting to communicate with the rest of the birth suite team, our midwife left the isolation room for the first time that night. She was going to talk to the doctors and plead for pain relief for me. She was deeply frustrated, distressed and understandably angry that our requests were being ignored.

After enduring another 4 hours of gruelling labour, I was in immense pain and I couldn't think how to relieve it, it just kept going on. Daddy paced the room anxiously, he seemed angry and knew he couldn't do anything being stuck in this room with me in agony. He even sought solace in a scalding hot shower, to sit and cry on the bathroom floor for a while. It was daylight now; I could see the sun peering through the steamed-up windows of our room that faced a lovely garden. The day was cold, and frost lay gently on the leaves of the tree, I focused on the glistening light while I was breathing through each and every one of those contractions. I remember this because it was going to be your birthday, a day and a night I will never forget. Soon a message came over the walkie talkie to say that they were ready to proceed with the C-section, that we had requested 7 hours earlier. You entered the world at 7:34 am. Despite the circumstances, you made your presence known with loud protests as they brought you into to our lives at the exact time, we had scheduled the C-section the day before.

Regrettably, immediately after receiving the spinal epidural for the C-section, I was suddenly struck with an intense headache that rendered me unable to think or function normally. I wanted to see and hold you, but I couldn't. My body was shaking uncontrollably, my eyesight went blurry, and I could hardly talk. Noticing I wasn't well, our midwife kept checking on me and asking the other doctors to help me., They gave me some more medicine to keep me calm. Despite all the people in the room that day, I felt profoundly alone.

When you, my beautiful son, were born and shown to us over the drapes, I couldn't help but feel overwhelmed by pain and sadness. Everything seemed interminably painful, as if it would never relent. Daddy was upset and overwhelmed with distress by witnessing me in such a state. That night had been long and filled with so many challenges. We were so overjoyed to meet you and to see that you were safe, but there was this profound sadness that this moment had to unfold under such difficult circumstances.

As you will learn later in life, Mummy had a condition called breast cancer long before you were born. To prevent further risk, I made the difficult decision to undergo a mastectomy, meaning I had to remove my breasts, so I wouldn't be able to provide you with breastmilk from my own body. We were so lucky to have a very special person in our lives, Serena, who generously provided her milk for you. I will forever cherish her kindness for doing this. We took some of this precious breastmilk to the hospital during labour and we asked for it to be stored in the hospital's fridge. Unfortunately, the milk was spoiled because it was not cared for. Our midwife had specifically asked for the milk to be stored in a fridge close to our birth suite so we could feed you as soon as you were born, but the milk was left out the entire time we were waiting for you to arrive, it was never placed in a fridge, so we couldn't use the milk that had been so kindly donated to us. We were mad and very sad that this happened. It was incredibly disappointing and disheartening that a significant amount of precious donated breastmilk was wasted and had to be discarded.

In these first few days and over the early weeks after your birth, I'm writing this letter to you and so I can preserve the memories of the journey to meet you. While I truly desire to send a letter to the hospital expressing our experience, I believe it's best to wait until I am stronger and have a better grasp of knowing how to care for you and to be a mummy. I need time to heal from the unexpected surgery we underwent, and to ensure that Daddy is doing alright too. He loves you as much as I do and we are both so overjoyed that you're finally here with us.

I want to make sure that you understand that I did everything within my capabilities to ensure your safety and nourishment while you were inside of me. I sang to you, read you books and Daddy and I danced together the night we were trying to bring you into the world.

I endeavoured to shield you from that nasty virus that was circulating, but unfortunately, it eventually caught up with me, the day you chose to arrive.

I'm Not Strong, I Am Surviving

I opted not to have the vaccines they recommend, believing it was the way to protect your health even if my decision was unconventional. Nonetheless, I stood by my choice.

I'm saddened that I couldn't have the birth that I had envisioned for us and I am sad that we had to experience meeting you in the way we did. But we are grateful to the special people that supported us to bring you into our world and that we have you to love and hold forever.

Love Mummy xx

I had worked over 14 hours straight that night with minimal food or water, I was in full PPE the entire time. I was not offered a break by other staff members, and I only left the room once to have a heated discussion with the doctor in charge, requesting pain relief for Katie and attempting to convince the night staff to take her to theatre for her planned caesarean section. I was overwhelmed, frustrated and felt I had let Katie and Jacob down, I felt like I hadn't protected them. Their experience of labour and birth was fraught with frustrations, fear and anger. After the birth of their baby in the operating theatre, and after many hours of arguing, fighting and advocating for the rights of Katie and Jacob, I returned to the birth suite, heavily burdened and tired. I stripped off my PPE, my scrub shirt and sat on the floor of the room we had occupied for all that time and I cried. The tears I shed were out of frustration for all that they had endured – the unexpected course of her caesarean section and the myriad of things she had been denied. My tears flowed mainly for what I couldn't provide her: the tranquil, serene environment she longed for, and the support she needed and deserved. I wept because our system made her feel insignificant, as if her needs didn't matter.

In the weeks following the birth of their son, Katie and Jacob engaged with debriefing sessions with me. The early days were distressing and challenging for all of us to navigate and process. Katie reported that she often woke up in tears, regretting the choices she felt compelled to make, and expressing how she felt pushed and pulled in various directions. Jacob at times during our discussions was visibly distressed, still grappling with witnessing what Katie went through that night. Despite providing his presence and support, he felt the sense of helplessness and hopelessness, believing he had not done enough or stood up. I, too harboured a lingering feeling in the pit of my stomach, wondering if there was more that I could have done. While I fought fiercely for them, I questioned whether I could have been more forceful for what she needed. I tried to engage with the doctors, I was respectful, partaking in discussions and making suggestions, but it all seemed to fall on deaf ears against the powerful system.

The road ahead for Katie, Jacob and their baby involved a long process of grieving and coming to terms with their birth experience. I encouraged them to write to the hospital, urging them to share their story and make it known what they were put through. It's unfortunate that so many women choose not to speak out, living with the agony and pain of birth trauma in silence. I wanted them to be heard.

Weeks later Katie wrote a letter to the hospital. She told me that she retold the story of her experience, asked for explanations and noted a few points that she felt were important to get answers for. She expressed their disappointment for the way both her and her husband were treated and mentioned the incident of her donated breastmilk being spoiled. She was even more disappointed in the response that she received several weeks later. She found it to be insincere and lacking adequate explanation for the treatment she and Jacob received that night.

There is an unspoken truth that the system 'grooms' women to conform to certain expectations, it subtly shapes women's experiences of childbirth. There is the fear, the language and the many outdated policies on how and when women should birth. I sometimes wonder, is it for the good of the women or for the good of the system? It is becoming more apparent to me that there is no trust in women's abilities to give birth, that labour can't initiate without interventions, and there is a large gaping hole where the support system should be for women to make informed decisions.

It is distressing to note that 1 in 3 women in Australia each year, experience some form of PTSD after giving birth. In a significant move, the state of New South Wales, has conducted the first ever parliamentary inquiry into birth trauma in 2023. This ground-breaking investigation received over 4000 submissions from women who had encountered various forms of birth trauma. Remarkably, these submissions included insights from midwives, nurses, doctors and other healthcare providers who either witnessed or were directly involved in instances of birth trauma or violence. The submissions allowed individuals to share their experiences while remaining anonymous if they chose to do so.

Not long after this incident, I found myself becoming increasingly fearful of the system I was working in. It sometimes felt dangerous to go to work, to work in system that was so broken. To not be able to support women, to increasingly watch the trauma, violence and damage happen right under my nose that I couldn't seem to make sense of or stop. I often felt that I had unintentionally caused harm while doing my job. There were numerous times when I questioned why certain practices or procedures were carried out and whether they were entirely necessary. I spent the days I was not working often replaying events in my mind, trying to find ways to explain to families why an intervention was done, or seeking allied health professionals to support the ones that were so fractured by the experience. I should have been able to enjoy my time away from work, like many others do, but the role I played in these traumatic births troubled me day and night. I frequently found myself defending my practice and in turn defending the empathy I held for the women in my care.

I have made mistakes and I am just going to hold them. They come in forms of uncertainty, in hope and in fear. I hear them repeating and try to ignore them.
I'll be patient and just hold on to them for a bit longer.

Chapter 15

Square Peg
Round Hole

Begging for forgiveness is a deeply harrowing and humiliating experience, one I have had to endure once in my midwifery career and am currently facing again. It honestly feels like being on my knees begging for my life to be spared.

Self-torment, anxiety, depression, doubts about competence and questioning self-worth all converge, leading to the overarching question – is it all worth it? The contemplation of whether to maintain my registration as a midwife looms large, and I've seriously considered surrendering it, eliminating the temptation to return.

I have teetered on the edge, close enough to feel the impending loss. The mental image of someone pressing the button on the computer to erase me from the system, never to resurface professionally, is a haunting thought. Surrendering my midwifery registration implies an irreversible step, a loss of identity. The title of midwife, worn with honour for so long, also carries a heavy burden of guilt and trepidation. I've questioned myself repeatedly – without it, who am

215

Midwife Crisis

I? What would I be if not a midwife? This internal struggle has been a defining and challenging aspect of my journey.

My journey to becoming a midwife and the path that led me to be the midwife I am today has been shaped by significant encounters, people, and by the women I have cared for. Waiting for the decision that eventually led to the restriction of my practice as a homebirth midwife, spanned almost 2 years, adding an agonising layer to this difficult process.

As I face another uncertain wait to hear what the system will decide for me now, it is important that I emphasise commitment to responsible practice. I am not dangerous or reckless, I am considerate and measured. I am dedicated to weighing up risks and prioritising the wellbeing of others. I consistently put the needs of others before my own; it's a deep level of compassion and respect for the women that I have worked with and cared for.

The establishment of a regulation authority in 2010 marked a significant shift in the regulatory landscape for health practitioners in Australia. Prior to this, registration was state and territory-based, meaning that practitioners were registered and governed by the regulations of the state in which they practised. The creation of the regulatory board consolidated all registered health practitioners under one national body.

While this move aimed to streamline and harmonise regulations, there are still variations in regulations and credentials across states and territories, adding complexity to the regulatory environment for healthcare providers. These variations are confusing and challenging to navigate for care providers, who may encounter different requirements in different regions. This still applies to private practising midwives across Australia, limiting their scopes of practice from state to state.

Square Peg Round Hole

The Nursing and Midwifery Board of Australia, in conjunction with the regulatory board, plays a crucial role in regulating public safety. They achieve this by developing guidelines, standards and codes of practice that set the expectations for the profession. Additionally, the board conducts investigations and takes disciplinary actions in response to notifications and complaints, ensuring accountability within the healthcare system. This comprehensive approach reflects the ongoing commitment to maintaining high standards and protecting the wellbeing of the public. I hold a large amount of respect for the work that is done and carried out by these boards. I also respect the codes of conduct and professional standards of practice.

Navigating a notification against you as a health practitioner is a challenging process devoid of practical guidance. Surprisingly, there is no comprehensive resource or roadmap for dealing with such situations. The fear of being reported to the regulatory board is a genuine concern amongst health providers, especially nurses and midwives, and namely private practice midwives, who find themselves frequently subjected to notifications and the experience remains distressing and daunting for those involved.

One aspect of the notification process is the uncertainty surrounding the timeframe for resolution. It's impossible to predict when the board will convene to address the matter. When navigating the process independently, without legal representation, individuals rely heavily on communication with case managers from the regulatory board. Keeping abreast of case managers can be difficult, as they change regularly and move jurisdictions.

In my personal experience, I endured a wait of over 12 months before being informed that there was no case to answer. Then, inexplicitly, my case was reopened, leading to another 12 months of waiting before homebirth restrictions were placed on my registration. Years later, as I am faced with yet another notification, I endure another long wait to hear my fate. The prolonged waiting periods prove to be the most challenging aspect, coupled with the emotional toll of having these notifications associated with my name. The sense of humiliation and shame that accompanies such situations is profoundly debilitating.

Belonging to the Australian Nurses and Midwives Federation (ANMF) proved to be an invaluable safety net for me as I navigated the daunting process of handling the notifications. Their unwavering support and acknowledgment of the immense stress involved were truly enlightening. I immediately contacted the ANMF once I was aware of the report against me and within a few days of receiving the notification, I was swiftly paired with a lawyer affiliated with the union, offered as pro bono assistance. This lawyer not only provided invaluable practical guidance but also advised me on the necessary steps and requirements to address the notification effectively.

During my latter years practising as a homebirth midwife, the development of the National Midwifery Guidelines for Consultation and Referral raised concerns among private practice midwives (PPM) caring for women outside the guideline's recommendations. There are many reasons why women choose care outside the system, and one glaringly obvious reason is the damage that has been done to women in such systems. The second edition sought to address these concerns by adding an appendix titled 'When a Woman Chooses Care Outside the ACM National Midwifery Guidelines for Consultation and Referral'. This guideline is useful and acts as a reference, giving guidance on how to navigate challenging circumstance when it comes to working with those that ultimately say no to recommendations. However, it is a guideline and can be at times difficult to apply to real-life situations.

A significant number of privately practising midwives are reported to the Nursing and Midwifery Board of Australia annually. A high percentage of these reports occur following orchestrated transfers from home to hospital, often initiated by the very healthcare facilities they are transferring care to. These transfers typically happen due to the need for further medicalised treatment, an intervention or emergency care. Personally, I received two notifications from facilities that I transferred to when I, as a private practice midwife, transferred care of women from home to hospital for continued medical care. Neither of these women gave birth at home. Our transfers were timely and appropriated, I was driven by reasons that warranted a transfer according to the guidelines, yet I faced reprimand for my actions. It often feels like a no-win situation, an ongoing battle between different modes of care.

I often seethe with frustration and anger at a system that seems to value policy and procedures over the very people it was meant to serve. In the sterile, bureaucratic maze of regulations, the humanity of my work as a midwife is lost amongst the policy and procedure. Each form, each protocol, was a barrier between the intimate, life-affirming care I have dedicated my life to providing. The faceless authorities, with their rigid adherence to rules, fail to see the profound impact of their decisions on real lives, reducing my years of compassion and skill to mere technicalities. The injustice of it all still burns within me, a constant reminder of a system that not only betrayed me, but the countless families I have served with unwavering dedication.

I have internalised much of my distress and suffering, presenting a façade of composure to the outside world. Over the years, I've carried undisclosed trauma that only recently became apparent to me. The trauma manifested in witnessing excessive blood loss, severe perineal tears, stillbirths, the language used to coerce women and regularly observing injuries sustained during instrumental births. Additionally, the notifications I have received triggered anxiety and distress, led me to re-evaluate my career choices and in some circumstances caused me to change the way I practised supporting women. It is, however, the enduring impact of witnessing women suffer the emotional pain and damage during birth, that continues to linger long after the notifications are closed. It became especially difficult to encourage women to make informed choices for themselves within the hospital system. The system is not designed to accommodate choices. As much as I wanted to fight for and empower women, it became an exhausting experience and somewhat a dangerous space (as I found out later) to be in.

In healthcare settings, the aftermath of adverse events tends to predominately focus on the patient. While their trauma, pain, grief and loss deserve and receive attention, there is a conspicuous absence of support for the individual/s who provided care for the patient. Psychological assistance for the healthcare practitioners within organisations is notably lacking. There is a continued emphasis on reporting the incidents that occur, with thorough reviews of documentation and prioritisation of what could have been done better. Adverse events are often used as examples of what would be done differently next time, and often used as learning experiences. Unfortunately, the wellbeing of practitioners is often overlooked and mostly disregarded in these scenarios. Practitioners who receive notifications against their practice following tragic or unexpected outcomes experience heightened anxiety and fear during investigations, which may lead to conditions being placed on or cancellation of their registration. Numerous reports and articles highlight the mental and financial stress that receiving a notification place on healthcare practitioners, pointing directly to the governing board of Australia's health service as responsible for this excessive burden. This board often fails to provide appropriate support during the process, leaving practitioners to arrange their own mental and financial support. In my research for this book, I encountered many stories of practitioners who took their own lives prior to or during investigations, not able to face the outcome of their fate. Not being able to manage the trauma, the shame and the guilt they faced after being involved in catastrophic events. Many were left with little to no support from their places of employment to manage the impact these events had on their lives.

I know the very same feelings of being left to fend for myself, scared and alone, being thrown into the deep end, without a lifesaving device.

Square Peg Round Hole

Seeking appropriate support is a challenging task. It can be very difficult to identify support services who can empathise with the profound stress, intricate details of our profession, the heavy weight of expected perfection at our job and the humiliation and panic that accompanies the role of a health professional that finds themselves under scrutiny. The practitioner may have crossed boundaries, practised outside their scope, or somehow been implicated in a tragic outcome. These events can profoundly shape health professionals, often becoming the focal point of their ongoing work. Practising under the constant fear of retribution or encountering a similar circumstance, is daunting and deeply impactful.

There is an expectation as a health professional to be an exemplary figure within the community. Being entrusted with people's health and wellbeing and engaging in ethical decisions in support of someone else's health, is a significant amount of responsibility to bear.

The guilt that I hold on to may never be resolved, but with time I am assured it will ease, and I will eventually feel safe enough to explore it openly with a professional that can provide me with a sense of clarity on it all. I struggle to comprehend the deep-seated feeling that resides in the pit of my stomach – perhaps it is shame. There is a sense of failure, a belief that I didn't execute decisions correctly and failed to meet the expectations placed upon me. Without appropriate supports in place within one's workplace, or without a safe place to address these feelings, it can be a lonely place to be. Overcoming the lingering sense of shame can be an arduous journey.

Looking back on the last few months as a caseload midwife, I now see that the prolonged hours, seemingly endless nights and weekends on call, and the trauma I encountered started to take a toll on my wellbeing. I regularly said yes and never said no, failing to create boundaries and failed to be aware of how this affected me and my own time. I worked behind the scenes on my days off, following up on results, responding to text messages, and offering advice and support. My work defined me, and my work ethic was such that I could only rest when the work was done – something that rarely happened. I was unable to rest, unable to get off the treadmill and allow myself to relax. I rarely slept a full night's sleep, even on days off. My nervous system was regulated to being available at any time, to get up and go, to constantly be on. I was always doing something that supported my work, whether it was studying, upskilling or attending conferences. Maybe I believed that the amount of work or study I did validated my worth within the workplace.

Complicating matters, I faced persistent challenges with the team manager, who felt compelled to scrutinise every action I took, every word I said, and every time I questioned a process. I was frequently summoned to their office to justify my decisions, explain the battles I had fought to advocate for a woman's choices, and then to defend my efforts to protect them against the system.

The term 'aggressive' was often directed at me. I had to be aggressive in my line of work, to defend and protect both myself and the women I cared for. If standing up for what I believe is right and not condoning inappropriate actions makes me aggressive, then yes, I was aggressive – and shouldn't everyone be? There were times when I was told I was too emotional and needed to take a step back. If being too passionate about my job and genuinely caring for my patients was a flaw, then they were right. I am dedicated to my role as a midwife and being with women means being fully committed to them. Advocacy for women and standing up for myself were consistent aspects of my approach to midwifery, but this stance ultimately became my downfall in many ways.

I don't want to be okay with the things I am no longer okay with.

Chapter 16

Speaking Up Can Get You Nowhere

Throughout my extensive career in midwifery, spanning many years and many workplaces, I have encountered a multitude of situations. However, never before have I found myself dedicating such a significant amount of time to defending, reporting and meticulously documenting incidents as I did during my tenure in hospital settings.

In a firm commitment to upholding standards of care and advocating for the wellbeing of the women that I care for, I once took a stand, reporting a particularly troubling incident. This experience has reinforced my dedication to ensuing the highest level of care for those I serve, even if it necessitates navigating the challenging terrain of incident reporting and documentation. Continuing my dedication to advocating for the rights of women whilst in the care of a healthcare setting. My goal remains rooted in promoting a safe, respectful and supportive environment for all individuals during their unique and transformative journeys, in the realm of midwifery. I am very passionate about speaking up for safety and for women to engage with health professionals on an even scale. In any setting be that of a workplace, a healthcare facility, a supermarket or a nightclub, no means no. We drum it into teenagers the need to gain consent, we ensure that even adults get consent to touch, fondle, kiss or hug one another. Gaining consent without coercive language to perform certain procedures or examinations in a healthcare setting should, therefore, be no different.

A pregnant woman should have autonomy over her body. It is her body, her baby and her choice. All healthcare professionals, regardless of their status, should respect the bodily autonomy of any woman they encounter. Women should be able to decline procedures in any setting, inclusive of the healthcare environment, without being coerced, threatened or forced into undertaking.

Gaining consent is a fundamental ethical principle that ensures respect for individuals' autonomy and decision-making rights. It involves clearly explaining the purpose, potential risks and benefits of a proposed action or agreement, allowing individuals to make informed choices. Effective consent requires the information presented in a manner free from coercion or undue influence. It must be voluntary, explicit and documented, ensuring that all parties involved have a clear understanding and agreement. This process is essential in various fields, including healthcare, research and legal contexts, to uphold integrity and trust in professional interactions.

Anita was a woman whom I had met during a stint in a suburban hospital. We met through the regular antenatal clinic I managed on a weekly basis. During these clinics I saw women who were in the early stages of pregnancy to those nearing the end of their pregnancies. I prescribed blood tests, planned and arranged their ultrasounds, monitored blood pressures, reassured them that the movements they felt were normal and ensured they were eating nutritious diets, to name a few aspects of my clinic day. I got to see the joy on their faces when they heard their baby's heartbeat and felt their baby kick under my hands as I palpated their tight, round bellies. I heard of their fears about childbirth, and I watched others cry reliving their past experiences. I met women I had never seen before and those that I had formed trusting relationships with. I offered each woman time to ask questions. I supported the hospital's policies, but also ensured they were aware of alternative options. I educated women, sharing relevant information that was evidenced-based and encouraged them to research and arm themselves with information to be able to make informed choices. This allowed us to make a care plan that supported her in choices in which she felt safe.

Preparing for her second birth, Anita was opting for a VBAC (Vaginal Birth After Caesarean) and we had discussed her plans and requests for this labour and birth at length. She diligently armed herself with information regarding the risks and best practices for VBAC. With no other risk factors and a normal pregnancy, Anita was confident and knew she had the right to make decisions about her mode of birth. She wanted to have the option to experience labour with minimal to no interventions. She explicitly communicated her decisions to me, which I had documented clearly. One of her requests was to avoid cervical examinations and to steer clear of stretch and sweeps prior to labour. A stretch and sweep involves a healthcare professional conducting a vaginal examination and attempting to sweep the membrane from around or within the cervix. While some believe that stretch and sweeps help induce labour, there is no evidence that this intervention alone can commence labour. Cervical examinations in late pregnancy can increase the risk of rupturing membranes (breaking waters) and increase the risk of introducing infection. I have performed these in my practice over many years, however I ensure that I have gained informed consent to do so without persuasive tactics and performed only when requested by the woman.

In her 41st week of pregnancy, Anita attended my clinic and had patiently waited almost 30 minutes past her scheduled time to see me, as my clinic was running overtime that day and she was the last person on my list. She was uncomfortable as during the last week of pregnancy her back pain had increased, and she was more than ready to meet this baby but was determined to wait it out if possible. Her demeanour was happy, she was always polite and friendly, and she was confident of her birth plan. It is normal protocol to offer CTG monitoring at least once a week past the due date, and Anita happily accepted the offer and went alone to the monitoring unit which was detached from the clinic. I had called ahead and was advised that she would be the last patient of the day. A CTG trace is where the fetal heart rate is measured by way of normal beat to beat, presence of variability of heartbeat and the reactivity of the baby whilst in utero. A CTG can detect any non-reassuring aspects of the baby's heartbeat and can be used to assess the wellbeing of the fetus. I assured her I would still be in the clinic when she finished and would review the results and let her know by phone, encouraging her to head home as soon as she was done. It was well past 6 pm when I received a call from Anita, distressed and crying. She told me the events that transpired in the monitoring unit in between her hysterical sobbing.

She arrived to see two remaining staff on duty. She was polite and chatty as she was strapped her in for monitoring. She waited comfortably for the monitoring to be completed. The CTG trace confirmed that her baby's heart rate was normal and that her baby was tracking well. As she prepared to leave, she was instructed to remove her underwear in preparation for an upcoming internal procedure. Confused by the assumption that she wanted an internal examination, Anita asked for an explanation, reiterating her clear preference to decline all internal examinations before labour. Despite her expressed wishes, her request was disregarded. Feeling intimidated, vulnerable, and too scared to argue, Anita reluctantly complied. During the call she had made to me, she expressed her experience as deeply disturbing and that she felt violated, as her requests were not respected. She had left the unit in such an emotional state that took her some time to calm down and to be able to drive home safely.

Speaking Up Can Get You Nowhere

I was not present during the incident, and I now wish I was, but I was very concerned by what had occurred. Anita was unable to recall who performed the examination but could adequately describe them to me. Approaching the monitoring unit, I was able to arrange a private discussion with the practitioner. The discussion I led emphasised the importance of consent for any procedure and I reiterated Anita's birth plan and her distinct request to avoid internal examinations. During this conversation, I was curious about how consent was obtained for the procedure.

It soon became obvious during the conversation that the practitioner understood the severity of their actions but believed the procedure was appropriate given Anita's gestation. It was evident that they misunderstood the significance of consent in this scenario. Frustrated by the lack of awareness of protecting and respecting women's rights within the system, I spent the next few hours reporting the incident. I then spent another hour on the phone with Anita, supporting and comforting her, and assuring her that I would ensure this would not happen again. I encouraged Anita to report the incident herself and, if necessary, to the police. Not wanting to cause trouble, she let me know she only reported the incident to the facility's complaints department that evening. And of course all of this was done outside of allotted my work hours for that day. I was rostered off that weekend but I could not let it go, I could not wait for this to be reported on Monday. I was focused on supporting and caring for a woman who had been violated and disrespected by a healthcare practitioner, in a system that was supposed to protect her.

A few days later, I found myself summoned to a manager's office, where another senior staff member was also present. Expecting a discussion focused on Anita's wellbeing, I was taken aback when the primary emphasis was placed on how I had approached the incident and how the discussion was perceived in the monitoring unit that day. Despite recounting the incident, my concerns for her welfare, and her explicit refusal of the examination, there was an astonishing lack of attention given to Anita's experience. This left me perturbed, heartbroken, and bitterly disappointed that this was not a woman-centred environment and that a woman's rights could be so easily disregarded.

I had spoken up for the safety of a patient, yet the focus remained on the perceived inappropriateness of my discussion with another health practitioner. I was told I did not escalate the incident properly, taking matters into my own hands was not appropriate and yet there was no acknowledgment of the gravity of the woman's distress or the protection I was seeking for her right to say no. Instead, I was asked to apologise for undermining another health practitioner's practice and for reporting the incident, which would leave a black mark against the practitioner. I adamantly refused to apologise, as it contradicted my principles and my respect for Anita and any other woman I provided care for.

In a disheartening turn of events, Anita received a tepid apology letter via email weeks later, which again fell short of addressing the core issue – consent.

It was a hard pill to swallow, and I began to recognise that the system prioritised protecting certain health practitioners over addressing incidents like this. It was simple: a woman said no, she did not consent to the procedure, yet she was coerced and ultimately forced to go ahead with something she did not want. This marked a turning point in my career, one I was not willing to ignore.

Let's not make women find their own reasons to not do what the systems say they should do; let's listen to why they don't want to do them and accept that.

Chapter 17

The Burn

I started to notice some signs of burnout gradually emerging – I didn't acknowledge them though. I stifled the feelings and I ignored the warning signs. I began to feel a sense of powerlessness, finding each battle increasingly challenging, and eventually I started to withdraw any extra efforts of providing care. I grew weary of constantly fighting and gave in to a few battles I just knew I wouldn't win. Advocating for women and their choices had been my life's mission; that was beginning to wane.

Weeks later I had noticed a slight resurgence after witnessing a few successful, pleasant births without any traumatic outcomes, I had not been summoned to the manager's office in weeks now and had been enjoying some well-deserved time off in between my on-call shifts. D and I had been planning an overseas holiday that we were eagerly anticipating. After another gruelling 13-hour day in the birth suite, I rode the elevator to my apartment, checking my emails on the way. There it was – the letter. As I read it, I felt that that old familiar gut-wrenching feeling. The words 'suspended for misconduct' echoed in my mind, leaving me in a daze. My head was spinning, I felt numb and was struggling to comprehend the implications of the suspension.

Midwife Crisis

The elevator arrived at my floor, and I couldn't move. I was frozen with fear. I re-read the first few sentences of the letter again. I slowly made my way up the stairs to my apartment door and fumbled with the keys to get in. Our hallway is long and dark, and I welcomed the darkness for the minute it took to reach the bright lights of the kitchen. D was in there cooking, the dog was barking loudly for attention, while I tried to catch my breath. The world continued on around me, but the pounding of my heart was deafening in my ears and the reality of what I had just read began to set in.

'How was your day?' D asked, his back to me at the stove.

'I just found out I have been suspended from work,' I managed to say slowly, putting my bags on the kitchen table. 'What does that exactly mean? And why?' he asked facing me, wooden spoon in hand. 'I don't know, I don't know what it means. But this email says I shouldn't come back to work until instructed to.' My voice was cracking. Panic rose in me. My heart began that all too familiar high-speed beat inside my chest. My ears began to ring and my throat went dry. What was happening? I could hardly string the words together. Hot tears welled up. I handed my phone over to D, so he could read the letter.

'Did you do it?' he asked after skimming the words on the screen. According to the letter, I had performed a procedure that was outside my scope of practice. While I was competent, qualified and experienced to carry out the procedure, the exact definition of a scope of practice, I was allegedly not authorised to do so in this health service.

As previously mentioned, and having worked extensively in private practice, continually enhancing expertise in different facets of midwifery is imperative. Over the years I devoted considerable time to educating myself in breastfeeding and lactation (however I do not practice as a lactation consultant), breastfeeding support and assisting families with babies who have various issues breastfeeding, including tongue ties. Additionally, I dedicated substantial effort to mastering the skill and procedure to revising anterior tongue ties. Through my involvement with an international association and collaborating with a seasoned practitioner who served as my mentor and evaluator, I eventually attained credentials in this field.

Despite the breadth of my skills, experience and credentials across various areas of midwifery practice, none of these were acknowledged or valued by the environment in which I was employed.

The reason for my suspension was that I had supported a woman in choosing a procedure to alleviate her baby's feeding issues. During the early phase of our postpartum care, we explored different options to address the situation. I referred her to other healthcare providers and presented alternative care options that were neither suitable nor available at the time. The woman and her partner, knowing and trusting me, aware of my credentials and experience, diligently assessed the risks and benefits of the procedure. They were pleased with the outcome, as their baby began to thrive, and their breastfeeding journey progressed successfully. My suspension did not result from any complaint from them; they were satisfied with my care and the procedure. Instead, it was imposed after another healthcare professional became aware of the procedure I had supported and carried out.

The letter of suspension instructed me not to contact my work colleagues or any of my caseload women. I was directed to call in sick each day of my suspension.

My colleagues, who were unaware of what had happened, were tasked with taking over my caseload in addition to their own. They were not informed of my sudden departure, and I was prohibited from taking phone calls or sending text messages to them. I felt ostracised and isolated from any support and I thought back to those who had received their marching orders during the pandemic; they must have felt the same. During this time, I was isolated from support and had no communication with my manager, as my phone calls and emails to them went unanswered.

During the suspension, I sought support from the ANMF (Australian Nurses and Midwives Federation). The ANMF team promptly responded, offering comprehensive guidance throughout the process. I was assigned a compassionate case manager who served as my voice of logic. She gently navigated me through each stage, assisted in drafting a statement, and patiently listened as I broke down over the phone on numerous occasions. Throughout many meetings and phone conversations with the ANMF teams, my credentials were deemed suitable and aligned with my scope of practice.

The representative from the ANMF provided unwavering support. She took over negotiations with the HR department, arranged the meetings I was required to attend, and guided me on what to say and how to say it. She offered emotional support, literally holding my hand and encouraging me to maintain my composure. She assured me that everything would be okay, but I couldn't shake the nagging feeling that it wouldn't be. To the first meeting, I wore black, feeling as if I were attending my own funeral. I felt numb and, for the first time in a long while, unemotional. I wanted nothing more than for it to be over. I had no desire to fight; I had nothing left to fight with.

During the meeting, we reviewed the events that had transpired. I was given the chance to respond, take accountability for my actions, and present my credentials. Although I remained composed, I was petrified by the confrontational nature of the meeting.

Throughout the 2-week suspension, I found myself in that dark and challenging headspace again. Each day felt like an eternity to come to an end and yet the nights were just as long and filled me with fear and sleeplessness, thinking and conjuring up what the next day would bring. For the first time in my life I began to take sleeping pills to help me through the nights and an anti-depressant to just keep my mind and thoughts in a less cluttered space. I saw a psychologist, but the darkness got heavier and harder to hold. I had felt this before, but this was different, it covered me like a thick, heavy blanket. This wasn't the person I knew myself to be – a motivated go-getter who loved her work. I struggled to make it through the day without breaking down. I felt like giving up. It was like I was walking through mud each day. The role I had once loved and thrived in for so many years, the identity I had formed for myself and what I had become, now left me feeling burned and scarred.

A simple road trip with D a few days after the initial suspension turned into a distressing experience. Nausea plagued me, and restlessness took hold as I sat in the passenger seat. When I took over my share of the driving, I was unable to concentrate. Every bump in the road triggered panic, causing me to grip the steering wheel so tightly my hands cramped, and fingernail marks were left in my palms. Eventually reaching our destination, I retreated to the hotel room. I didn't attend the function we had come for, drawing the curtains, needing to shut out the world and the humiliation I felt.

I had been explicitly told not to contact any of my work colleagues, but I was unable to continue the façade and reached out to Ruby letting her in on what had happened. We then met regularly for coffee and lunch dates where I would spend most of the time distressed and unable to control my emotions. Unleashing my fears and worries, she gave me space and time to talk, reflect and express my feelings. She held out her hand to me kept me above the water. My lifelong friend Rachael became my saviour during this time, the sunshine I needed that I had begun to shut out. She provided me with the tenderness and care I craved so badly at the time. I was devasted, I was uncomfortable and embarrassed at the situation that I had found myself in. She reminded me that I was worthy and capable, reminding me that I would resurface after this was over, no matter what the outcome. I feared for the repercussions of the suspension, which filled me with dread. I received no support, mental or emotional, from my employer. I took on the accountability for my actions but yet there was no duty of care from them and especially in this era of mental health awareness. It is still very difficult for me to comprehend.

The final decision came in the form of an email, asking me to attend another meeting where they would discuss their plan of action on the 14th day of my suspension. It was both a relief that it would soon be over and also a tidal wave of emotions of what I would be facing. I had already decided to resign from my position, as the humiliation and possible consequences were not acceptable to me. With the assistance of my union representative, a resignation was negotiated instead of a termination, which had been their decision. I declined the face-to-face meeting where they planned to present this, preferring to take control of my exit with some semblance of dignity. I was not offered an exit interview; instead, I was requested to return my work equipment in person. The journey there for the last time was incredibly difficult and distressing. I was filled with anger and fear, and the mere thought of running into someone I knew or a colleague caused me to shake. I was in no state to be pleasant or explain my absence to anyone that day.

The main reception through the car park is a wide area surrounded by glass walls and a glass ceiling. On a cloudless day, the sunlight is blinding and reflects a rainbow of colours on the walls. However, as I stepped out of the lift that day, the space felt dull and lifeless. It was raining and the grey sky muted the usually colourful entry. Under the neon sign that illuminates the institution's name, logo and establishment date, stands a large wooden plaque. Carved out of wood in the shape of a wave, it proudly reads: 'WE VALUE EVERY PERSON – WHETHER PATIENT, THEIR FAMILY OR CARERS, AND ESPECIALLY OUR STAFF'. I stood staring at that plaque, noticing it for the first time. It felt as though that wave was rolling towards me, ready to wash me out. The HR manager, whom I had met once at the initial meeting, greeted me with a fixed smile, glancing up at the sign I stood beneath. With a nod and a gesture to follow her, we stepped into the elevator in silence. She led me through a maze of dimly lit corridors on the top floor to a small, stale, secluded office. As we walked, I noticed that no other offices we passed were occupied. She handed me a pre-prepared checklist of equipment to return, then coldly thanked me for coming in and handed me a parking voucher, asking if I needed an escort out. I was shocked and confused at this approach and naively I had assumed she would enquire about my wellbeing. Instead, it felt like a robotic procedure, where I was merely processed as another statistic. It left me feeling marginalised, as though I was being treated as a criminal rather than a once-valued employee. This was striking and contrary to the anticipated care and consideration you would expect from such an organisation that prides itself on values such as compassion, hospitality and respect. Walking back through those corridors to my car, I passed that wave sign again, feeling bemused and shocked by what I had just encountered. It entirely contradicted the institution's proclaimed values.

In the days following my resignation, I felt I could breathe a bit easier and almost began to relax. I didn't feel that tight wound-up feeling, I slept well, ate meals at normal times, and enjoyed the break from on-call work. I spent time exercising, cooking and taking trips I hadn't normally been able to take. I made arrangements to see friends without the fear of being called into work and was able to do simple, everyday activities. I began applying for other roles and had been successful in job interviews. I was just starting to regain my confidence.

Then, of course, the storm rolled in, and everything quickly unravelled when I received a call from a case manager at the regulatory board. That old feeling crept back inside me, even before the case manager finished explaining the reason for the call. The hospital had filed a notification against me, outlining allegations that would be emailed to me the following day. I was told I would have 14 days to respond and was advised to contact a counselling hotline if I found this distressing. There was that token approach to support again. Not only had the hospital planned to terminate my employment, but they had also initiated a misconduct case against me, deepening my sense of betrayal, humiliation and shame.

It was a month after my resignation and learning of the notification I was to face, D and I took a reflective and restorative trip overseas. We immersed ourselves in healthy activities, swam, spent time in the sun, travelled to new places, and began to reflect on our lives, both as a couple and as individuals. During this break from reality, I started musing about this book. Although I was still wounded, scarred, fragile and broken, I needed to remind myself that I was worthy, that I was a good and careful midwife, and that the title did not define me.

I was uncomfortable with the predicament I had found myself in, but I needed to begin to uncover the wounds, tell the story of how I got here, and start to re-establish myself. I had done it once before, and I could do it again. The notification still loomed over me, leaving me uncertain about my future and whether I would hold on to my registration. I was exhausted thinking I would have to go through this again, trying hard not to think about my past, present or future.

Once again, I reached out to the ANMF, who appointed me a lawyer (pro bono) to support and defend my case. We worked tirelessly together, gathering evidence of my credentials. I prepared a statement and attended required courses. I acknowledged the boundary I had crossed and began preparing myself for what lay ahead and the worst possible scenario.

The following months were filled with waiting and uncertainty. I even seriously contemplated surrendering my registration. Naively, I had trusted the system to protect me, assuming it would provide support. However, I found myself alone, forced to fight and wait once again. My confidence wavered, and the passion for being a midwife, or the midwife I had always been, soon became tainted, stained, and too painful to contemplate as my future anymore. I

The Burn

am a conscientious person, never intending to hurt or harm anyone. Throughout my career, my focus has been on providing support, guidance and trust, and the highest level of care. Despite going above and beyond, I find myself facing the repercussions of not fitting inside the box and straying beyond the lines.

As I write this my fate remains uncertain, and the outcome of the notification against me is still pending, leaving me in a state of limbo. Despite the challenges and my mental turmoil, I currently maintain my registration as an endorsed midwife and have not chosen to surrender it. This period has compelled me to reflect deeply on my career, my practice, and all the circumstances that led me to this predicament.

At times I have questioned whether the issue was with me, feeling that I didn't align with the values of the maternity system and institutions that uphold it, and that maybe I was a misfit – a square peg in a round hole. However, through this ordeal, I have come to realise that I am perfectly suited, inherently round, but I have been trying to force myself in that rigid square hole for far too long. It is time to exhale, release the tension and embrace the authenticity that comes with being true to myself.

Keep going, keep providing, keep
caring and keep shining.

Chapter 18

This is Going to Hurt

While writing this book I contacted the Nurse and Midwife Support Service. I was reluctant because I had attempted to access their support in the early days post the loss of the homebirth baby many years ago. I was distraught and desperate for help. I had no-one to talk to about my feelings around what I had been through and the hurt I had inside. The shock still hadn't worn off and I was drowning in my own grief, all the while pretending to be a strong, independent midwife that could just carry on. I had other women to care for, women who were relying on me to be their midwife. I had a business to run and a family to manage as well.

The Nurse and Midwife Support Service was a new enterprise at the time and like most new businesses had some teething issues. The calls and the emails I sent went unanswered for weeks, and when I was eventually called back, the person I spoke to on the phone was unable to help me. It seemed my concerns and requests for support were not able to be met. They hadn't dealt with private practice midwives before. I lost faith in the service and wrote them off. Funnily enough, I do recall referring students and other midwives to their services back then.

Midwife Crisis

Recently, I gave them another go. By this stage they had developed an arm of the service that specifically helped nurses and midwives who were dealing with notifications. They had called it Notification Navigator, which seemed fitting for the purpose of their service. I was matched up with a consultant called Carol. Carol and I now speak regularly. She understands my distress, listens and lets me tell my story. We talk regularly about the theory of moral injury that occurs more regularly amongst healthcare providers who are involved in or witness traumatic events.

While I seldom receive direct answers from her regarding the issues that have arisen in my career, I do find solace in the substantial support and resources she provides.

Carol and I recently discussed an article she had read, outlining why midwives are particularly vulnerable to PTSD. It truly resonated with me, and I questioned if we even know that we get PTSD from the trauma we witness day in day out. The sessions I had with her were relaxed, our conversations flowed easily and many times I let go of my stress. She made me comfortable to talk about my situation, the issues that plagued me and I learnt so much from her.

As facilitators of birth, midwives are regularly exposed to distressing and confrontational scenes in the birthing space. Despite the emotional toll, many midwives put on a brave face, solider on and shake off these experiences. This resilience is often maintained, despite the turmoil going on inside. There is an expectation for midwives to be brave, rock-solid and return to work the very next day after enduring trauma, and to be ready to face similar scenarios once again. It soon becomes a normal aspect of the role, to regularly see excessive blood loss, fetal demise, fetal death and even generalised trauma and assault on women's bodies. Midwives endure these challenges with little or no support, minimal recognition of the trauma they experience from their workplaces and are often given flippant references to workplace counselling services. The absence of sufficient support systems compounds the emotional strain experienced by midwives in their daily work.

Exposure to regular traumatic experiences undoubtedly renders midwives vulnerable to what is known as vicarious trauma.

In the realm of midwifery care, there exists a profound sense of guilt and responsibility toward the birthing women. The relationship that a midwife forms with a woman in her care is unlike any other in the healthcare industry, particularly in models of continuity of care such as caseload and private midwifery practice. Alongside this responsibility, midwives commonly experience a range of emotions such as grief, anger, confusion, withdrawal and flashbacks to traumatic events. These feelings are inherent to the nature of the work and can manifest as a result of the challenging experiences encountered during labour and birth.

Students who accompany women through their pregnancy, birth and postpartum journeys are also exposed to this type of trauma, as they become deeply engaged with the woman throughout the process. Without adequate support, these students may perceive such trauma as a normal aspect of midwifery practice, rather than recognising it as the result of the interventions that cause birth trauma. Therefore, it is crucial to provide comprehensive support and resources to both midwives and students to navigate and mitigate the effects of vicarious trauma.

In the birth space, midwives frequently find themselves in a situation where they are expected to compromise their values and belief in women's birthing abilities. They often witness a disregard for women's requests or needs, disregard of a woman's rights and commonly witness neglect to obtain consent or the provision of biased opinions. Inappropriate language is not uncommon in the birth space, and midwives may feel pressure to comply with institutional policies and procedures that don't respect or align with the woman's wishes. This can serve as a significant catalyst for the moral distress or trauma experienced by midwives in various settings.

In my 2-decade long career, I've encountered a spectrum of diverse birth experiences. I've been privileged to witness the serenity of blissful births in unconventional settings like lounge rooms, bathrooms, on toilets and even in hallways. I've also had the opportunity to support, and guide frightened, traumatised women towards empowered births that they never thought they would achieve. From assisting first-time mothers to multigravida women, I've journeyed alongside women through the entire spectrum of pregnancy, birth and postpartum, an honour I have never taken for granted and will forever hold close to my heart.

Throughout this expansive career, I have recognised significant disparities between homebirth and hospital birth. Having worked in both capacities – as a homebirth midwife and a hospital birth midwife – the contrast is striking. With homebirths, I had consistently felt secure, composed and equipped to navigate the unknown, whereas the atmosphere in hospital births often left me feeling apprehensive, unsettled and unprepared for unforeseen circumstances. Despite the common perception that a midwife's role remains consistent regardless of the setting, my experience has revealed otherwise.

We know it all works out,
eventually. Know that everything
happens for a reason and
everything has a season.

Afterword

Fate Unfolded

A pregnancy typically lasts 9 months or so. I have supported many that went longer than this but that's the generalised expected timeframe for human gestation. Similarly and ironically, it took 9 months and 3 days for the second notification against me to be resolved. Those 9 months were, in many ways, similar to a pregnancy. My days often started with a nauseating feeling. I was fatigued, I experienced emotional fluxions, I had physical discomfort and many moments of intense anxiety. And much like a first-time mother awaiting labour and birth, I found myself consumed by the fear of the unknown. Waiting. Uncertain whether I would receive a reprimand, a conditional decision or a complete revocation of my registration. I often imagined the worst-case scenario and contemplated its implications for my future.

I initially harboured some scepticism about the experience of the lawyer that had been assigned to represent me in the case of practising outside my scope. Our interactions were solely through phone calls or emails, and I had never met her in person. Her mannerisms and voice appeared youthful, which raised doubts in my mind throughout the process. She quickly reassured me that my concerns were unfounded. She approached the situation with directness, providing clear instructions on navigating the notification with professionalism and poise. While her demeanour lacked emotion and empathy, I recognised that her job and the role she was trained to do was so starkly different from my own.

Responding to a notification typically involves extensive documentation, including submission of credentials and evidence of and competence in the field as well as any completed training. Additionally, individuals may be obligated to undertake various courses or compose a reflective assignment addressing the allegations. This assignment prompts individuals to contemplate alternative actions, acknowledging any mistakes made, review their decision-making, practice or consider how they would approach the situation differently. Despite completing all these tasks diligently, I couldn't shake lingering questions: was it all worth it? Was my time up now? How could I ever return to the profession? In what capacity could I return? Would I ever return to practising as a midwife?

Following the submission of all necessary documents, including a reflective piece on my actions that felt akin to pleading for forgiveness, I found myself immersed in a period of waiting. Each day was filled with anticipation for the decision that would ultimately shape my future, determine the trajectory of my career and the continuation of my journey in midwifery. The waiting period was challenging, and uncertainty loomed large, casting a shadow over every aspect of my professional life. Applying for jobs became a daunting task, overshadowed by the fear of not knowing whether my midwifery registration would be affected, whether restrictions would be imposed, or if I would retain my registration at all. I began to write this book with vengeance. It took all my concentration; it consumed me and it reminded me of what I had to offer and what I was worth.

The call finally came from the lawyer on an ordinary Thursday, her phone number always appearing as a No Caller ID. Home alone, I picked up the call tentatively, and just hearing her voice on the other end sent shivers down my spine as I held my breath, anticipating the conversation. She was not one for small talk and with no break after our initial greetings, she launched right into it.

'You have no case to answer. We will close the case now. You did a good job on the submission. Congratulations,' she said, her tone calm and concise, devoid of emotion.

'What does this mean?' I asked, feeling as though her words weren't quite real, questioning if I had heard her correctly.

'It means that they don't see you as a risk, that your practice *was* within your scope, albeit not at *that* institution, but you are now cleared. There will be no conditions or reprimand on your registration,' she explained, her voice almost rising with excitement. I thanked her for her part in the successful case, and she even asked if I was okay. It struck me, I had rarely ever been asked that question throughout my career. Teary and shaken I said I was. I was in disbelief, relieved and suddenly as though the huge weight that had been crushing me for the longest time had finally been lifted from me. I felt as though I had been released from something that had held me down for a very long time. I could breathe again.

In the weeks after resolving the notification and realising I could continue my career as a midwife, I began to slowly unwind. My tormented mind stopped racing, and the pounding in my ears ceased. My heartbeat returned to a normal rate and I didn't jump in fear when the phone rang. I stopped judging myself and slowly started to accept the enormity of what I had been through.

One of the hardest truths I had to face was that, regardless of the outcome, it was unlikely I would ever be the same midwife I once was. The midwife I had been could no longer exist in this world; the system didn't want her and wouldn't allow her to be who she was. Sometimes, our greatest strengths can become our greatest weaknesses and vulnerabilities. So now the love story is over, and I

Midwife Crisis

am as heartbroken as anyone would be after losing the love of their life. When you seek love, you desire safety, passion, support, and trust. Believe me, that's all I ever wanted from the career I chose, and it's all I ever gave it.

I'm letting go now, with love and grace, honouring the midwife I once was but will no longer be.

I looked at my old life one last time, taking a deep inward breath, I held onto all that I had achieved, all that I had done and I gently told myself, this is it, this is the time. You are ready for your new storybook to begin.

About the Author

Kelli is a highly experienced midwife with a passion for providing exceptional care to women and their families. She was one of the first graduating students of the Bachelor of Midwifery in Victoria, Australia, and has since accumulated a wealth of knowledge and experience in various healthcare settings.

Throughout her career, Kelli has worked in both public and private hospitals, where she has had the opportunity to support and guide countless women through the journey of pregnancy, childbirth and postpartum care. She has also worked as a private midwife for an OB GYN, offering personalised care and attention to expectant mothers.

In addition to her hospital-based work, Kelli has made significant contributions to indigenous health. She has worked in indigenous health centers, running clinics and programs specifically designed for young indigenous mothers and their babies. Her dedication to improving maternal and child health outcomes for indigenous communities has been highly commendable.

Starting her own private practice midwifery centres was a highlight of her career forging the way as one of the first to hold an endorsed midwife status, including becoming a Medicare eligible midwife. Her private practices included homebirth services where she could support women and their partners to choose birth in a safe holistic environment.

Midwife Crisis

Kelli's expertise extends beyond her work as a practitioner. She has also served as an educator, sharing her knowledge and experience with aspiring midwives. She has worked at SIDS and Kids Australia as an educator, raising awareness about safe infant sleep practices. Additionally, she has served as an educator and practice support midwife at Canberra University in the Bachelor of Midwifery program, mentoring and guiding future midwives.

Outside of her professional endeavours, Kelli is a loving mother of two adult sons and has been happily married for almost 30 years. She is a true entrepreneur at heart and has successfully operated other businesses including a shoe boutique and a café.

With her wealth of experience, dedication and compassionate approach, Kelli is a trusted and respected midwife who continues to make a positive impact on the lives of women and families in her community.

Gallery

Midwife Crisis

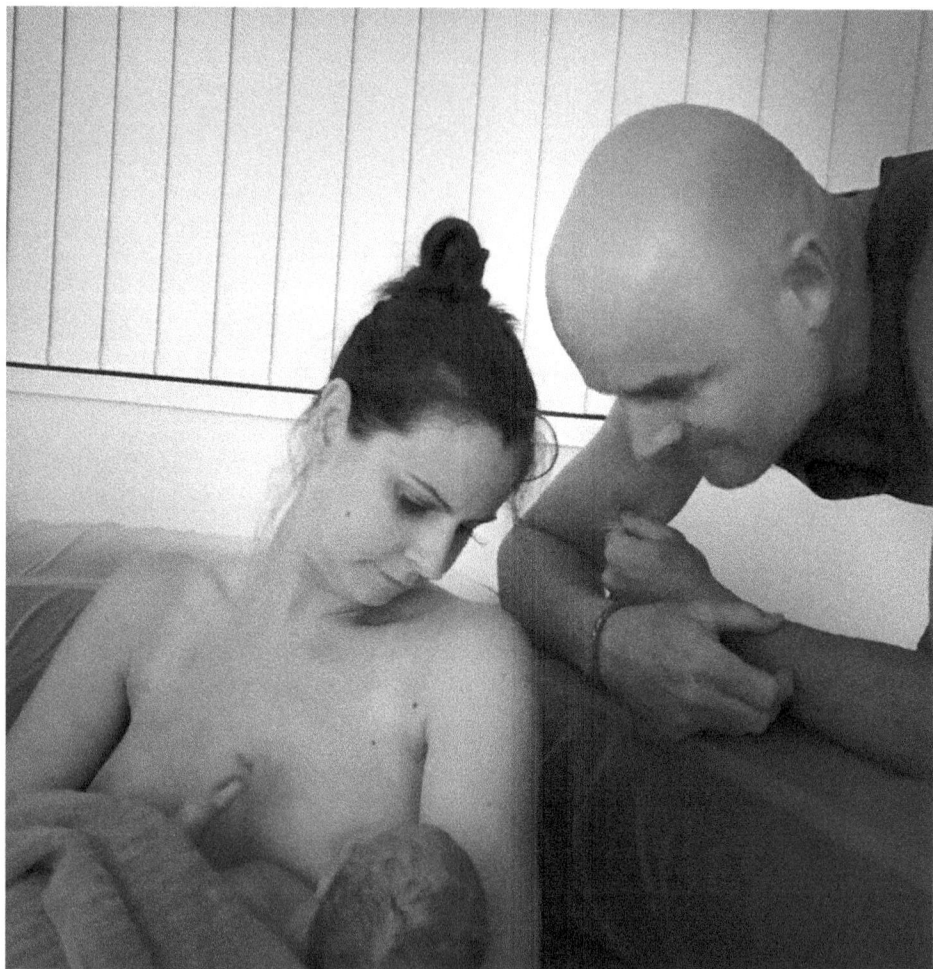

Gallery

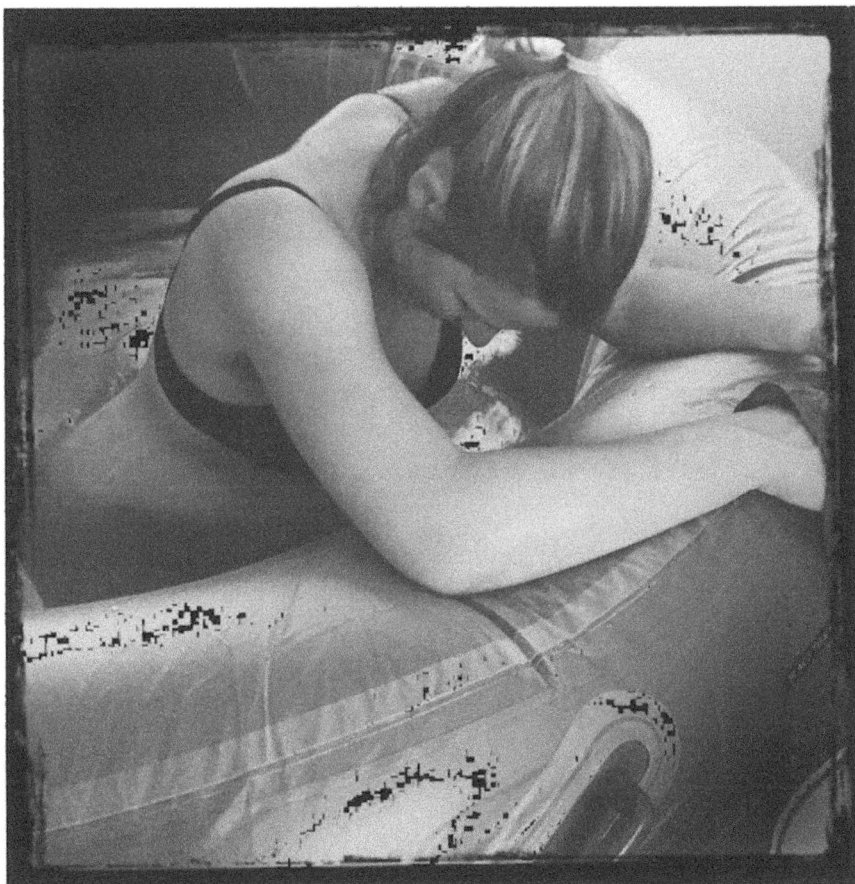

AUG   16

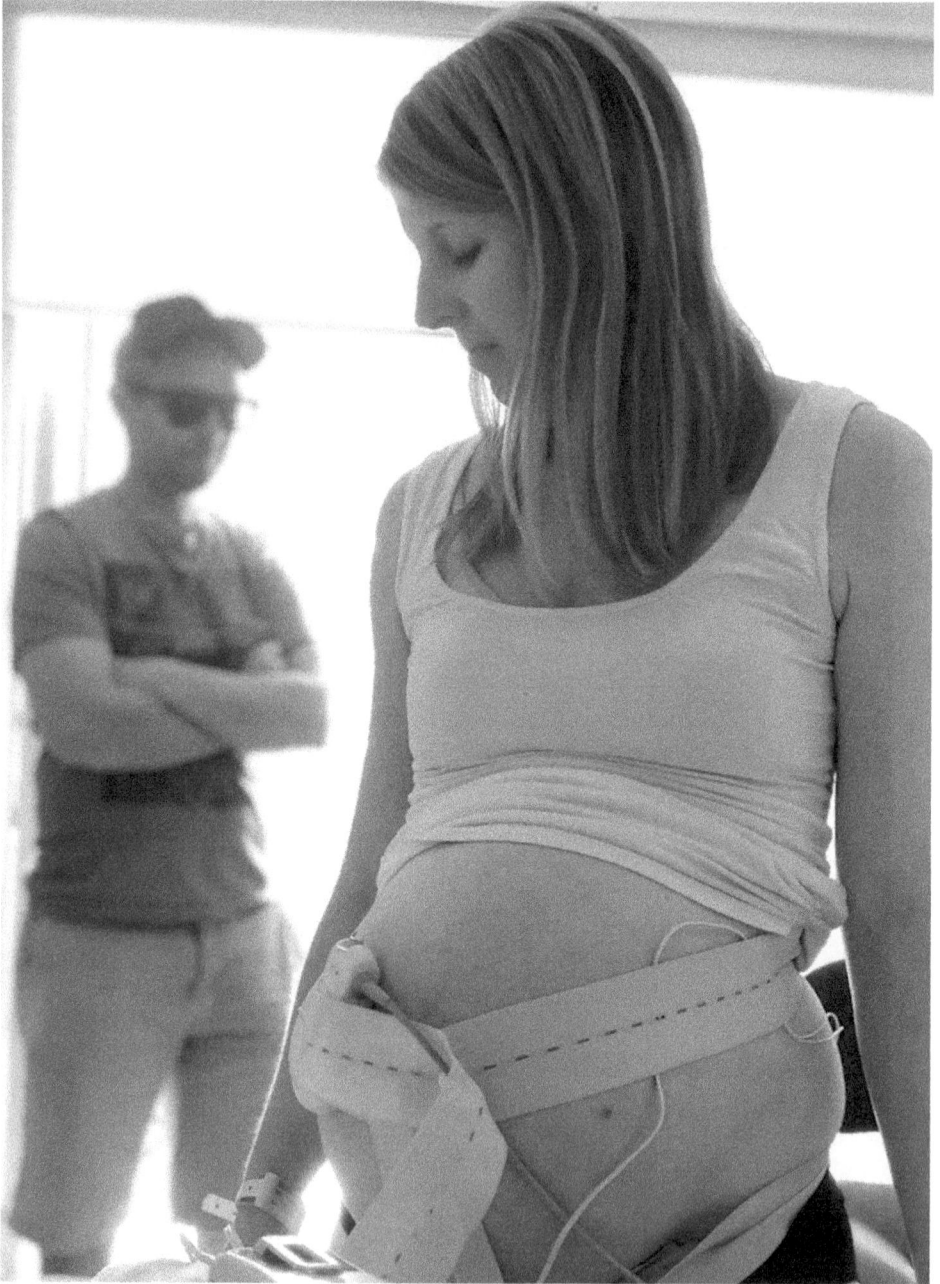

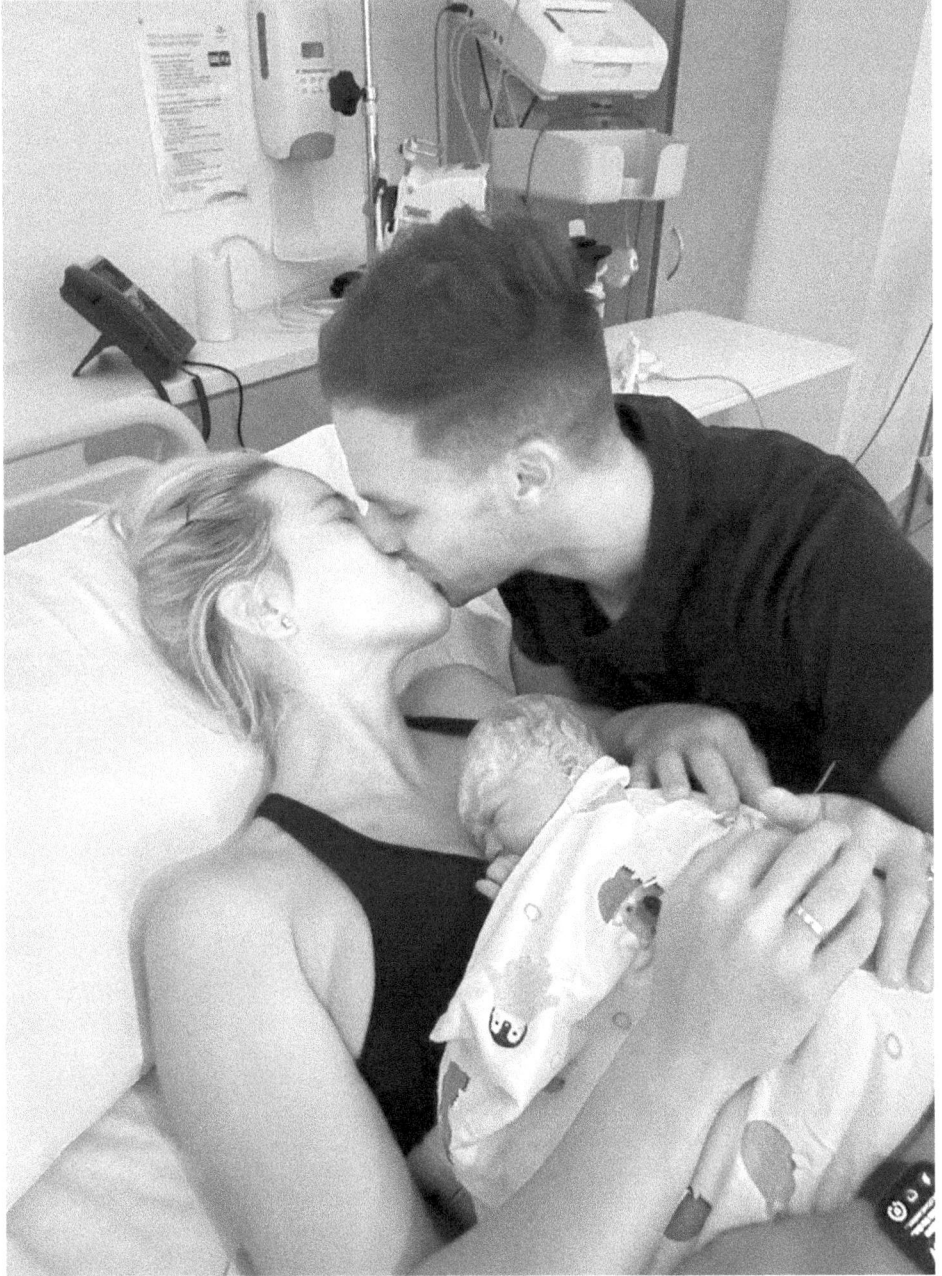

Midwife Crisis

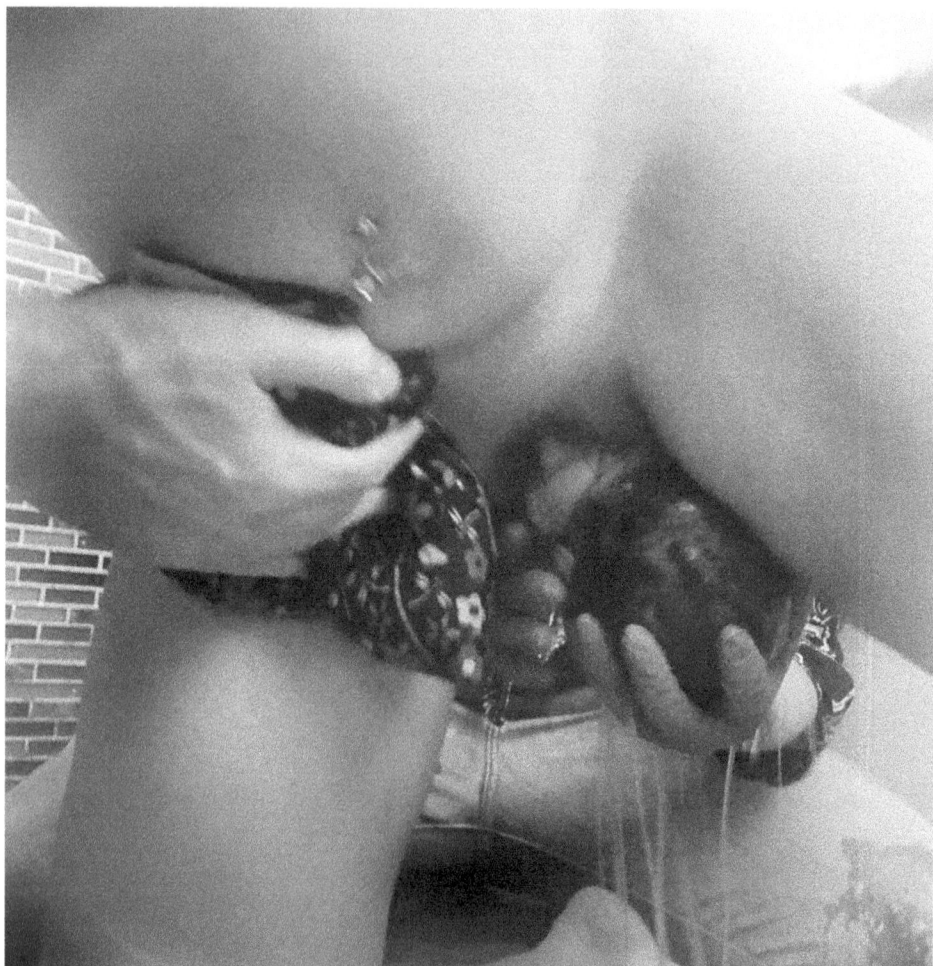

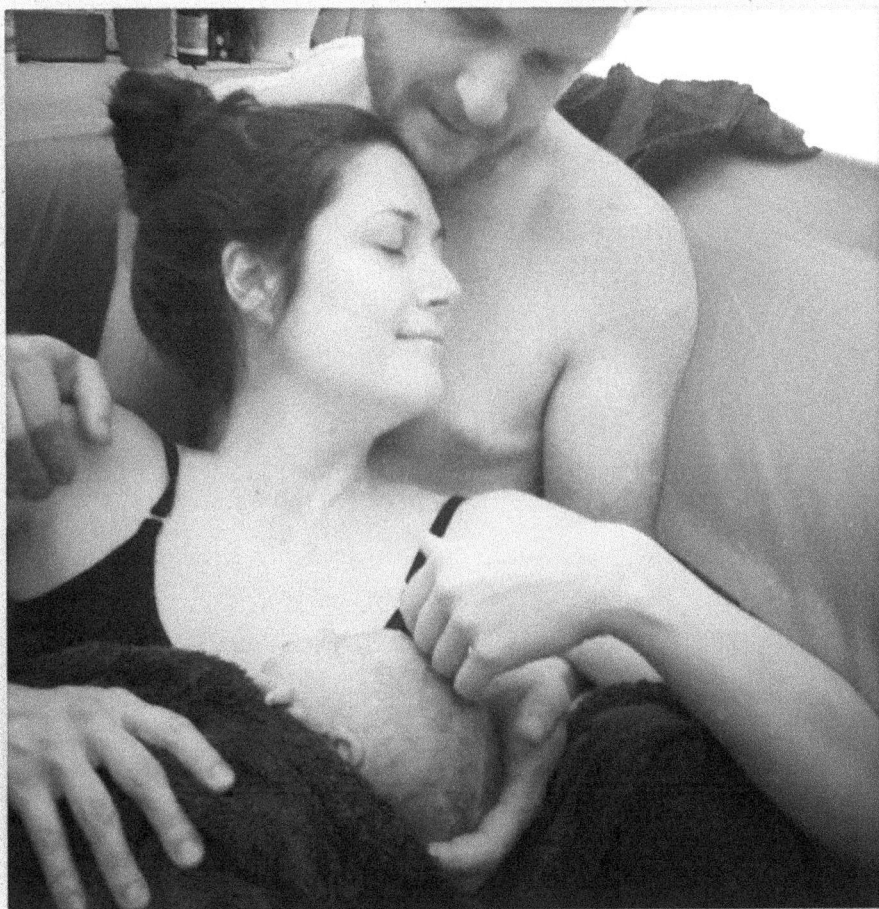

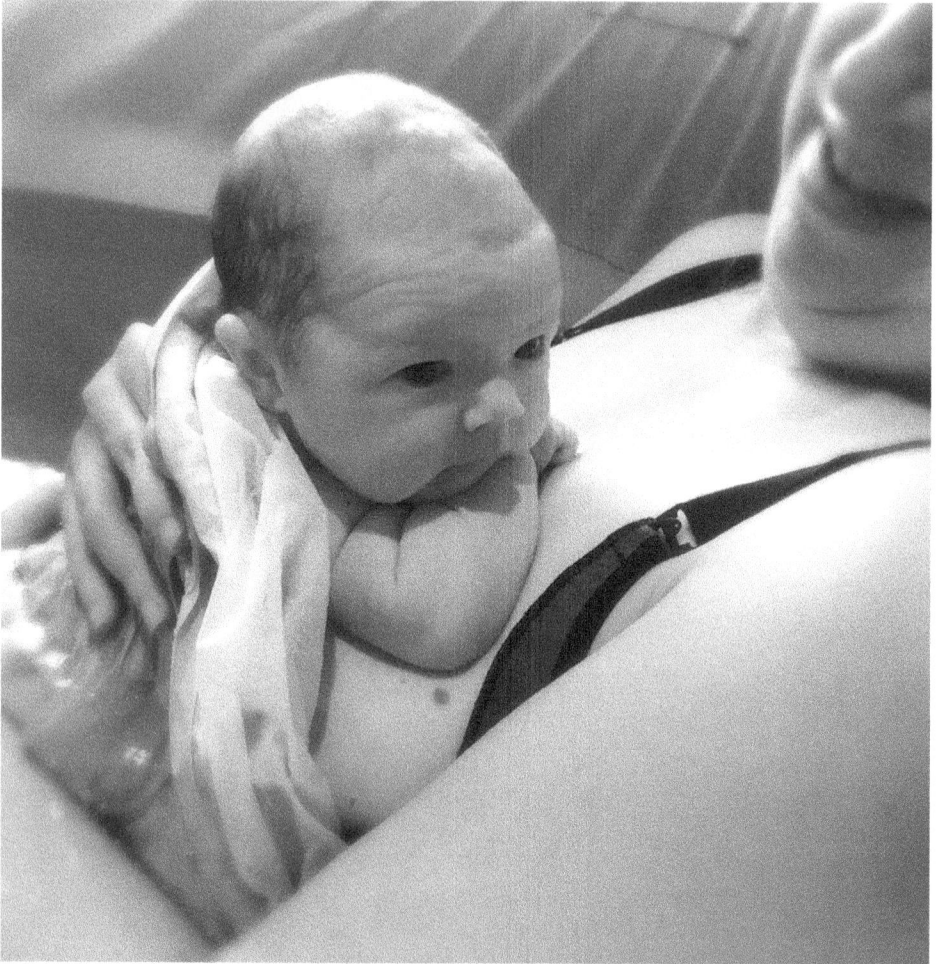

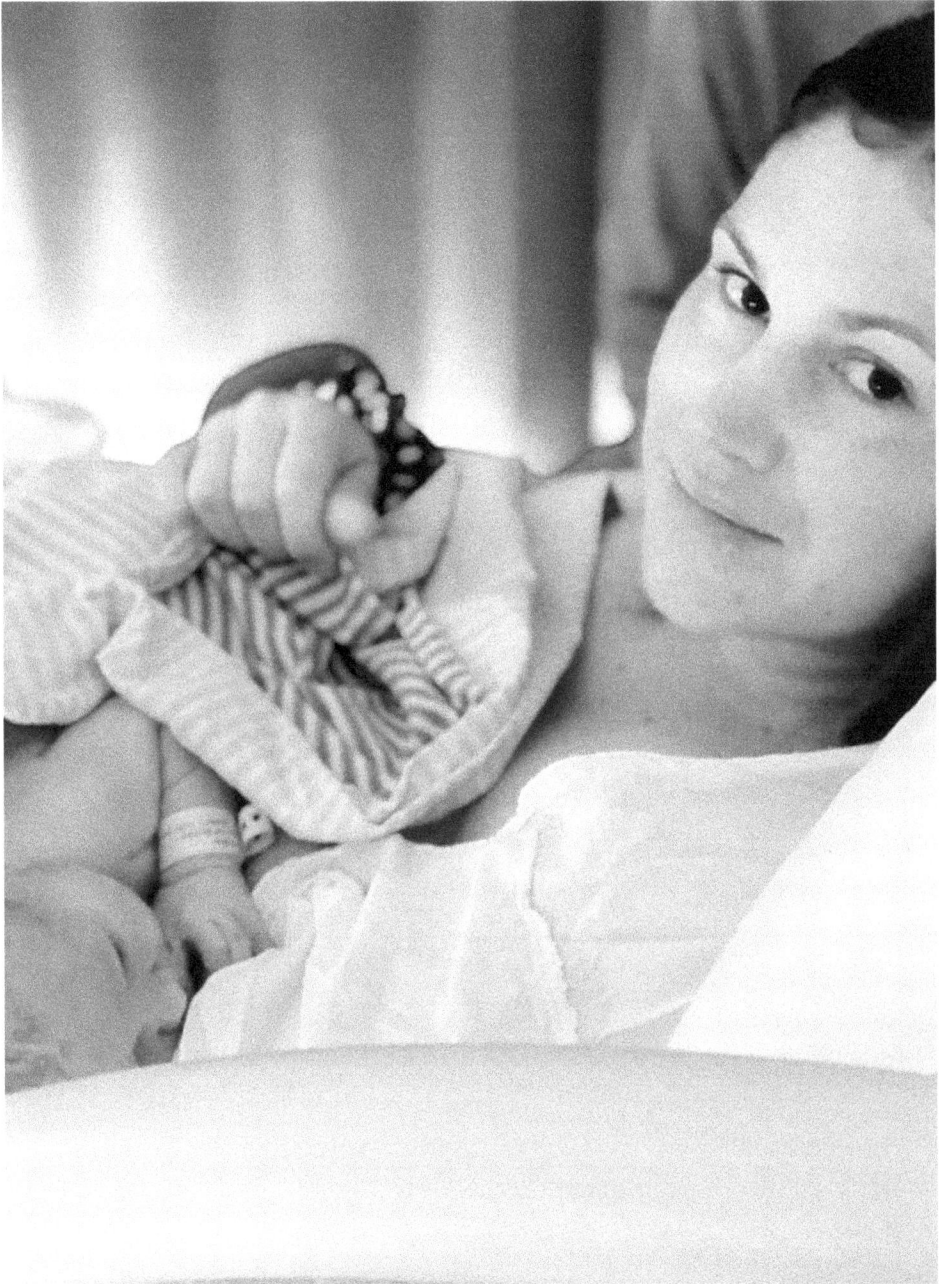

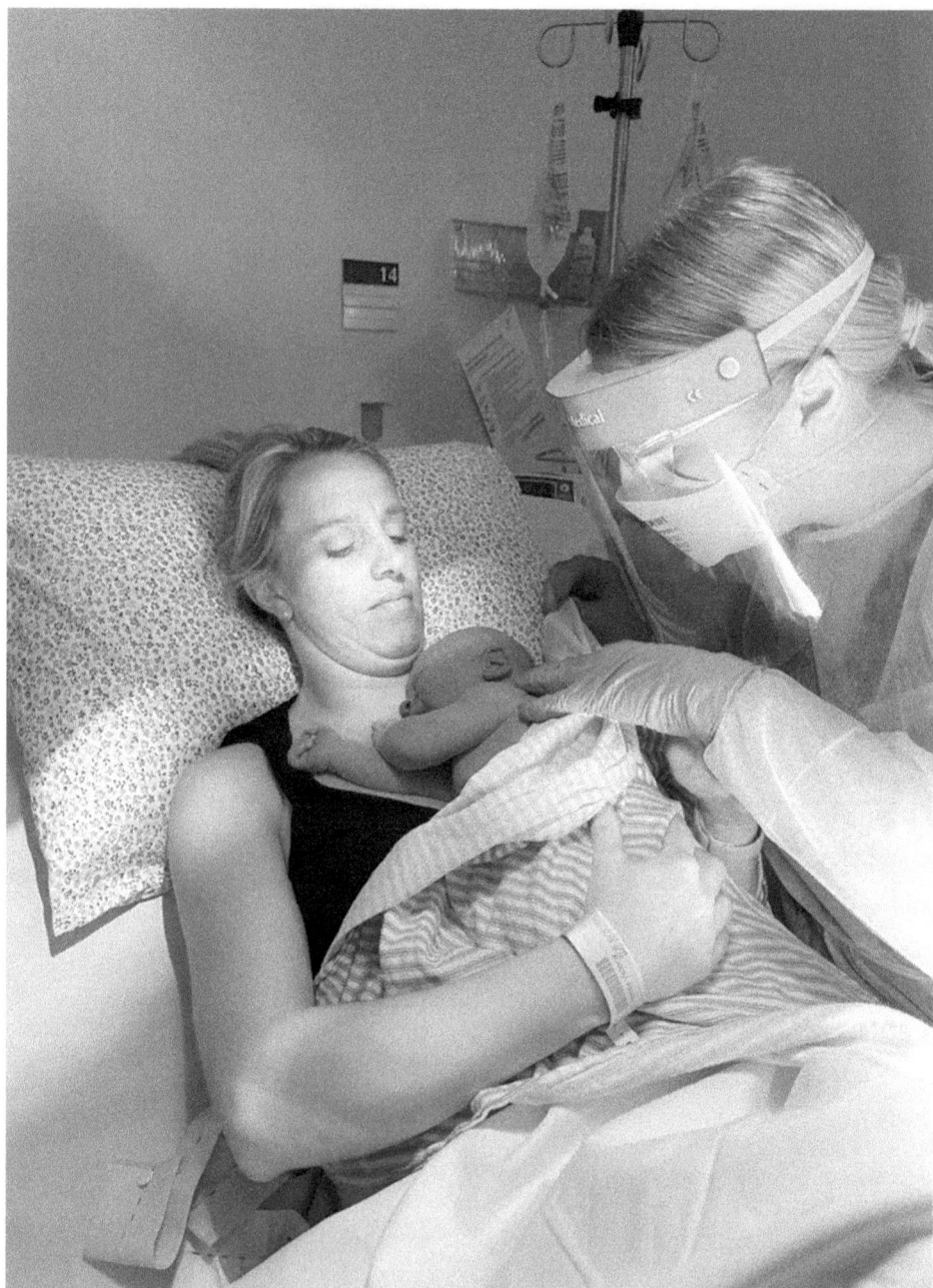

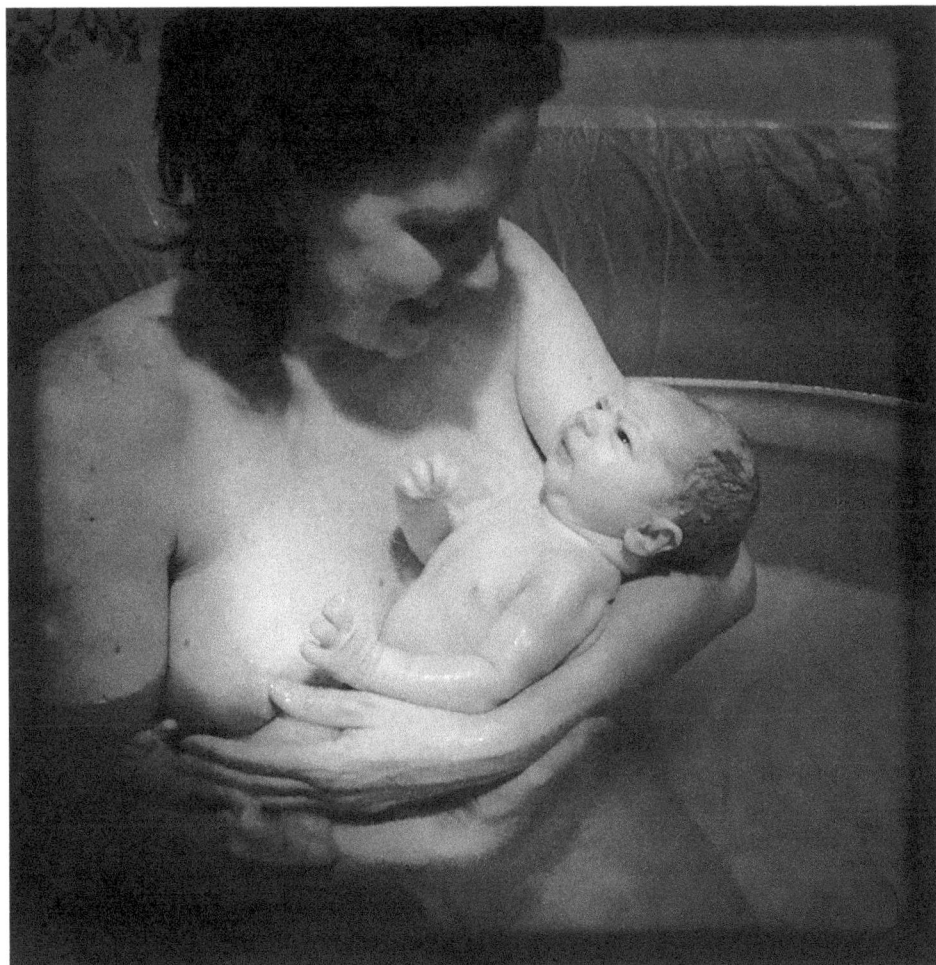

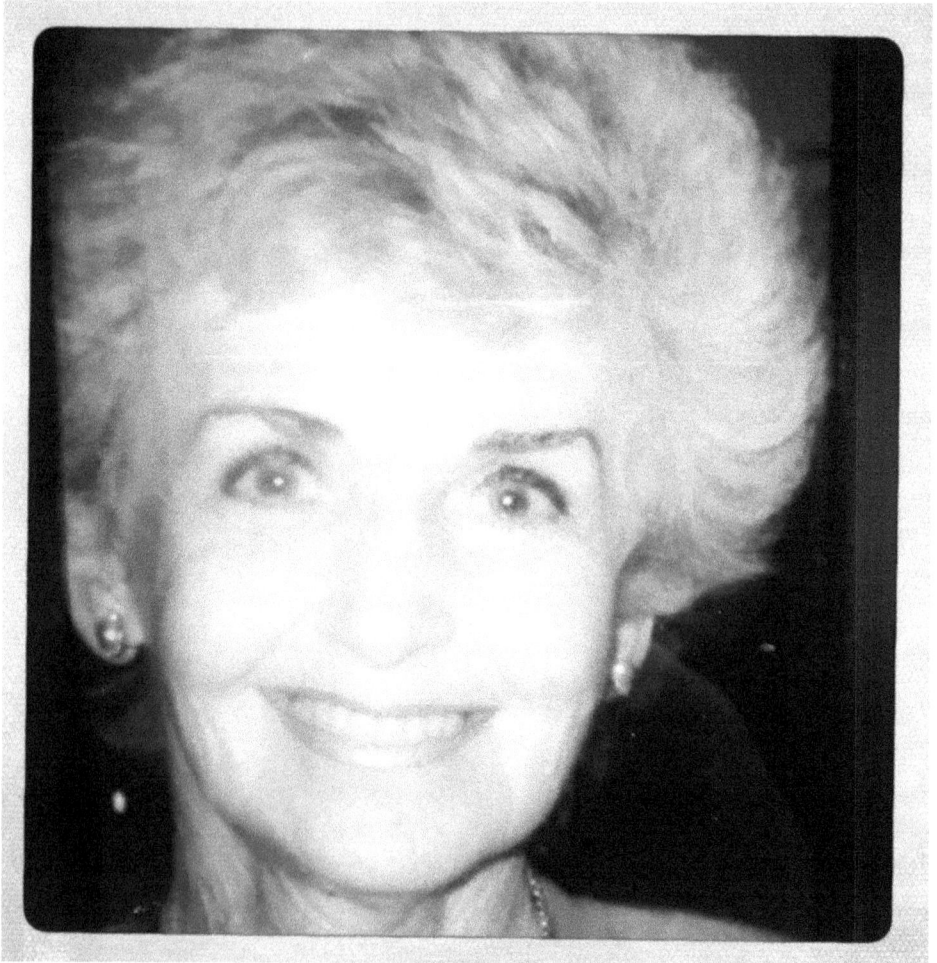

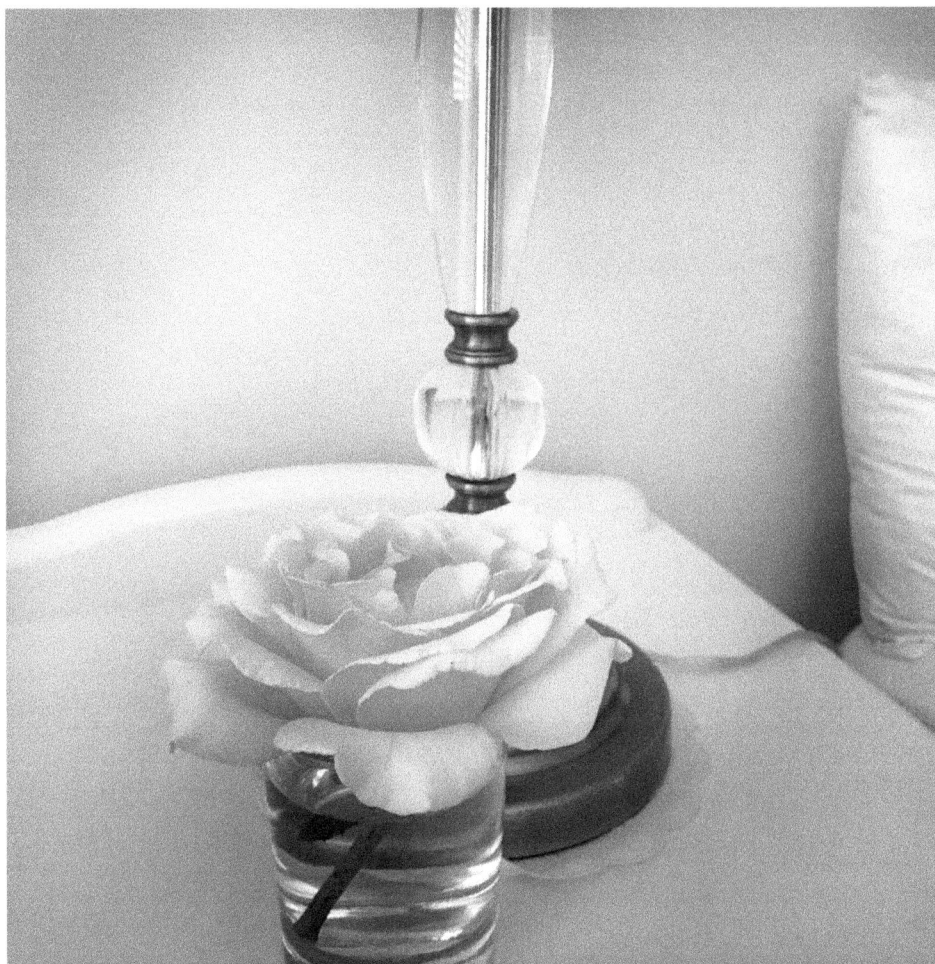

Midwife Crisis

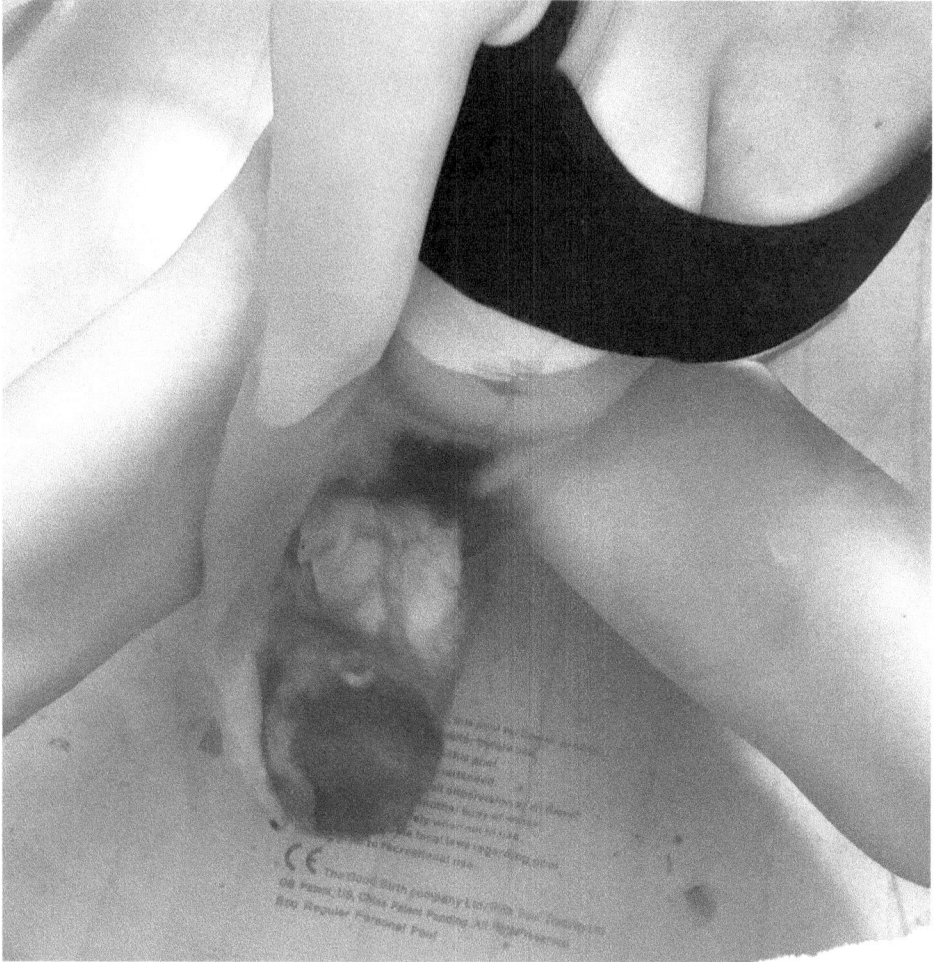

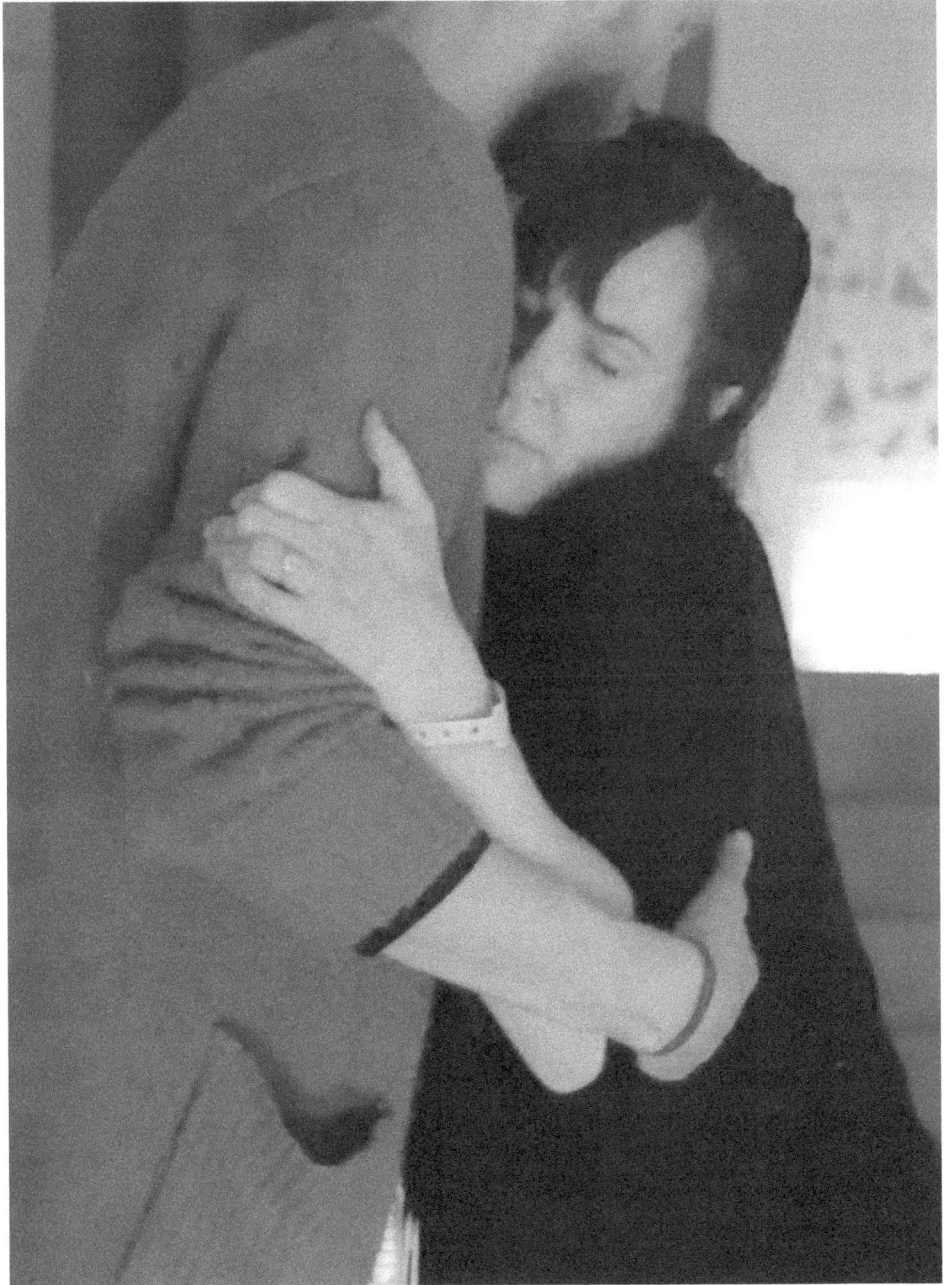

Midwife Crisis

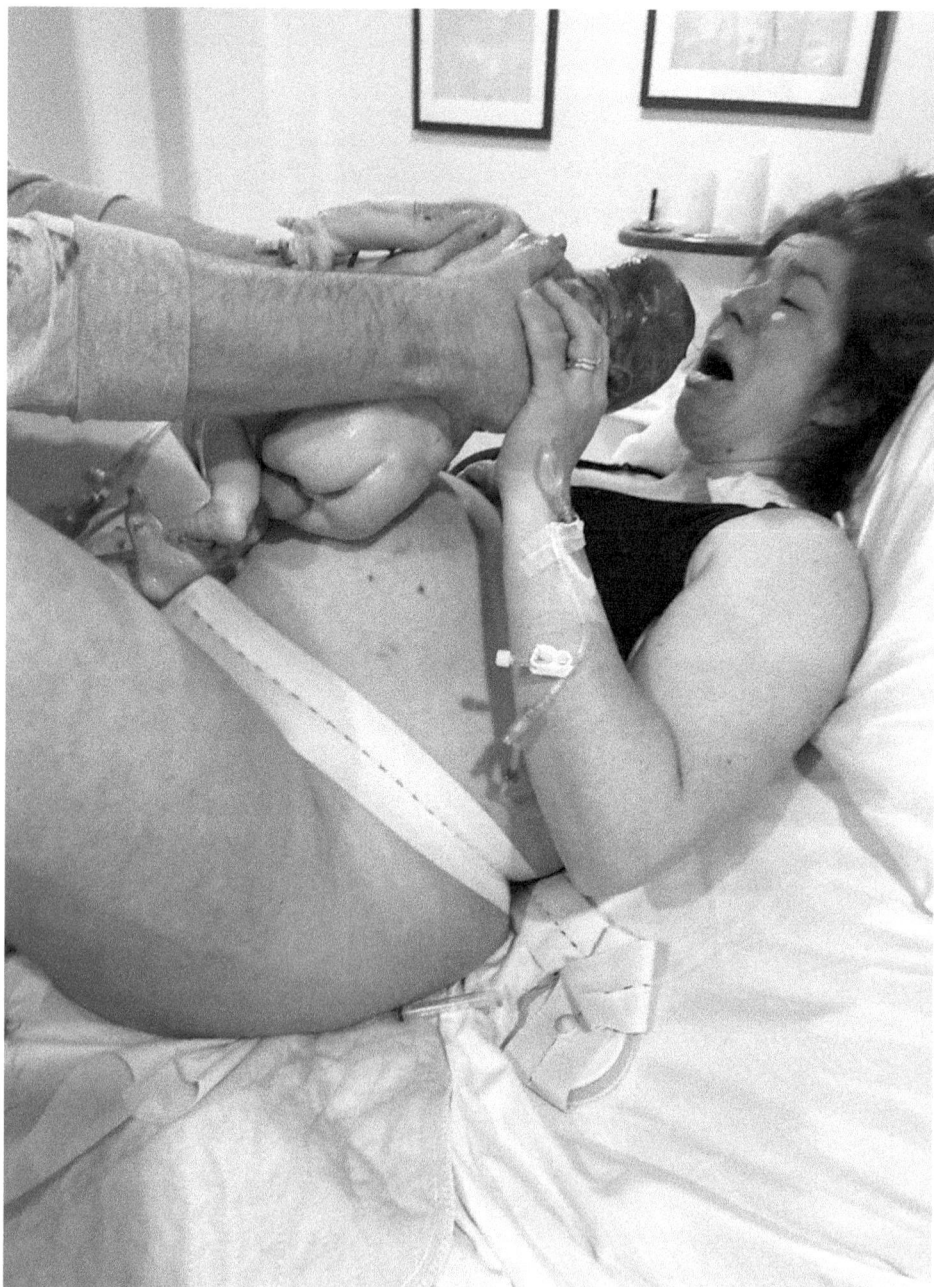

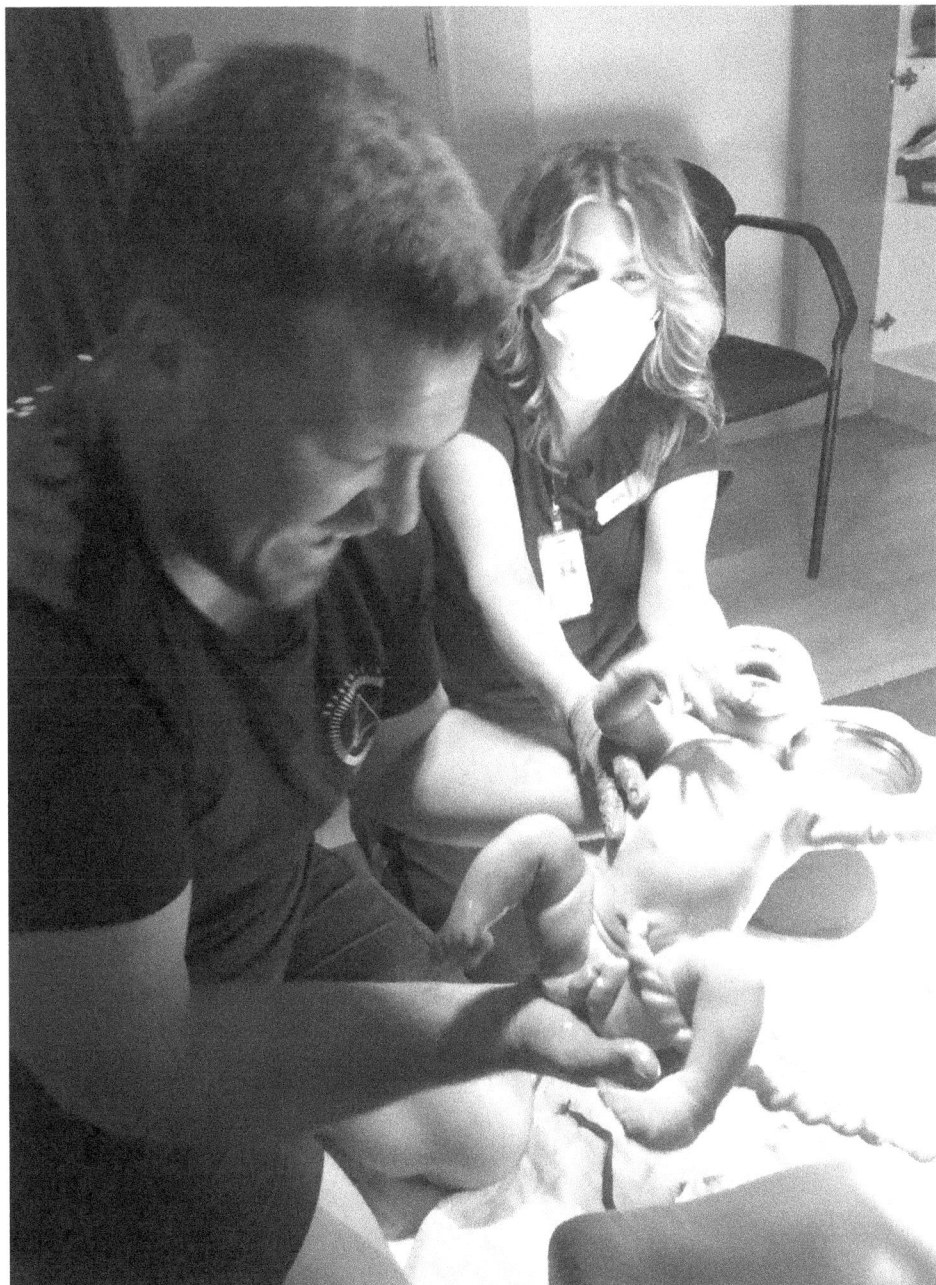

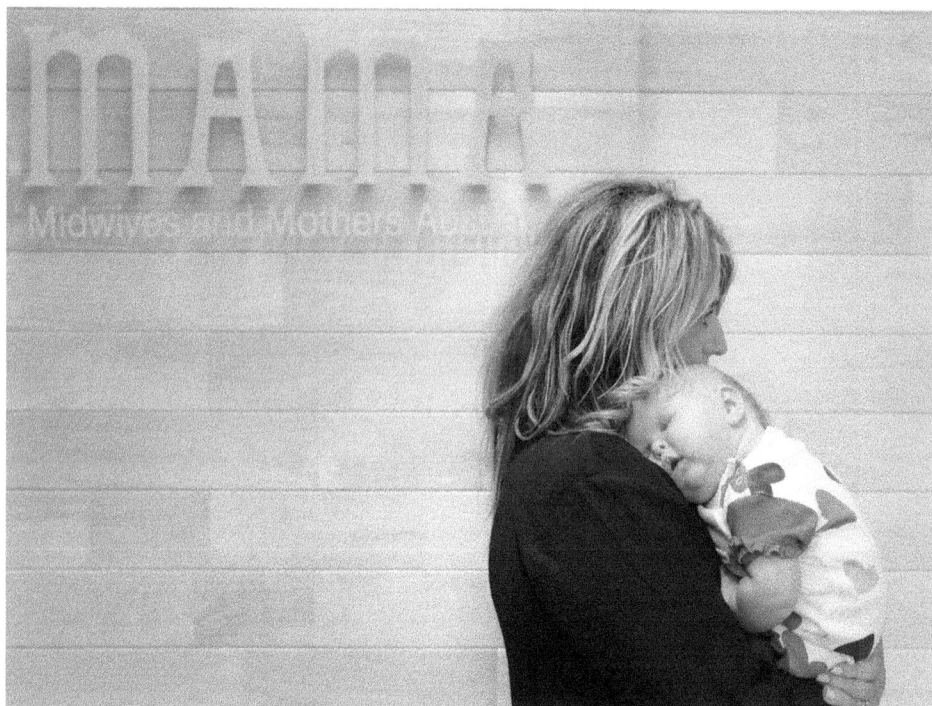

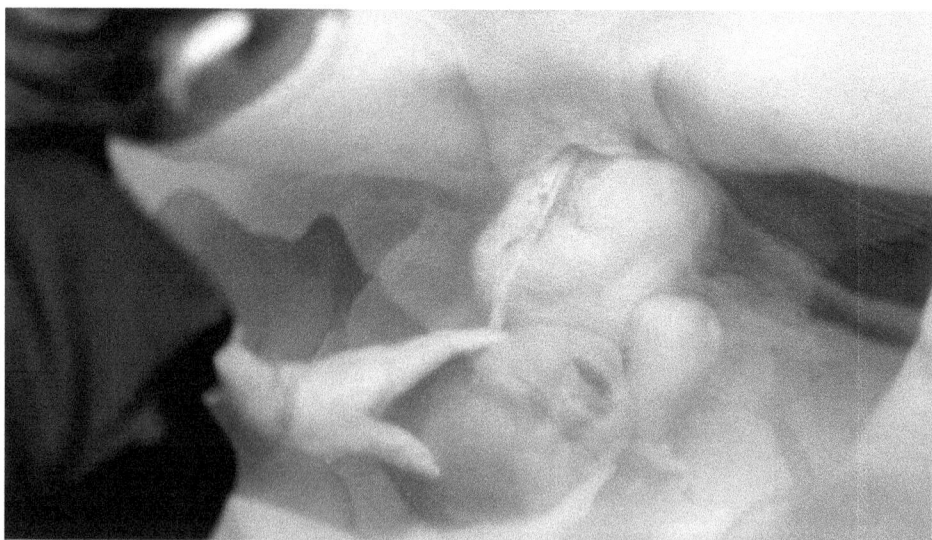

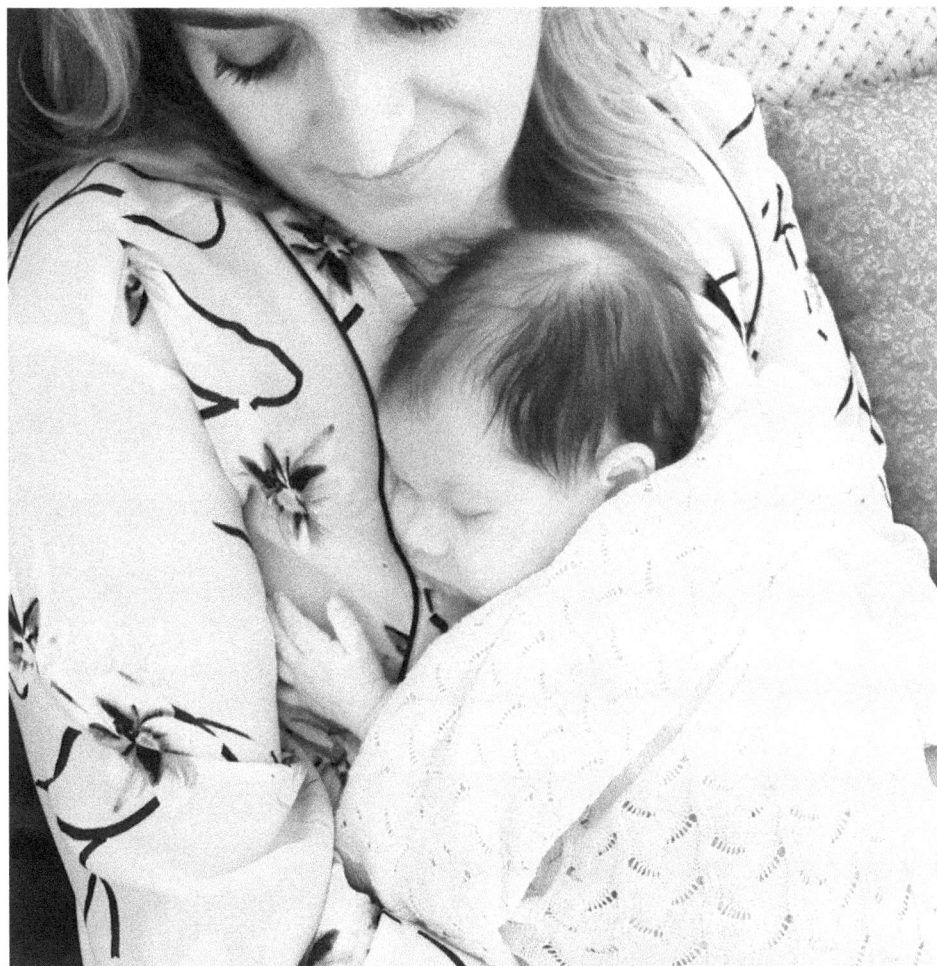

Midwife Crisis

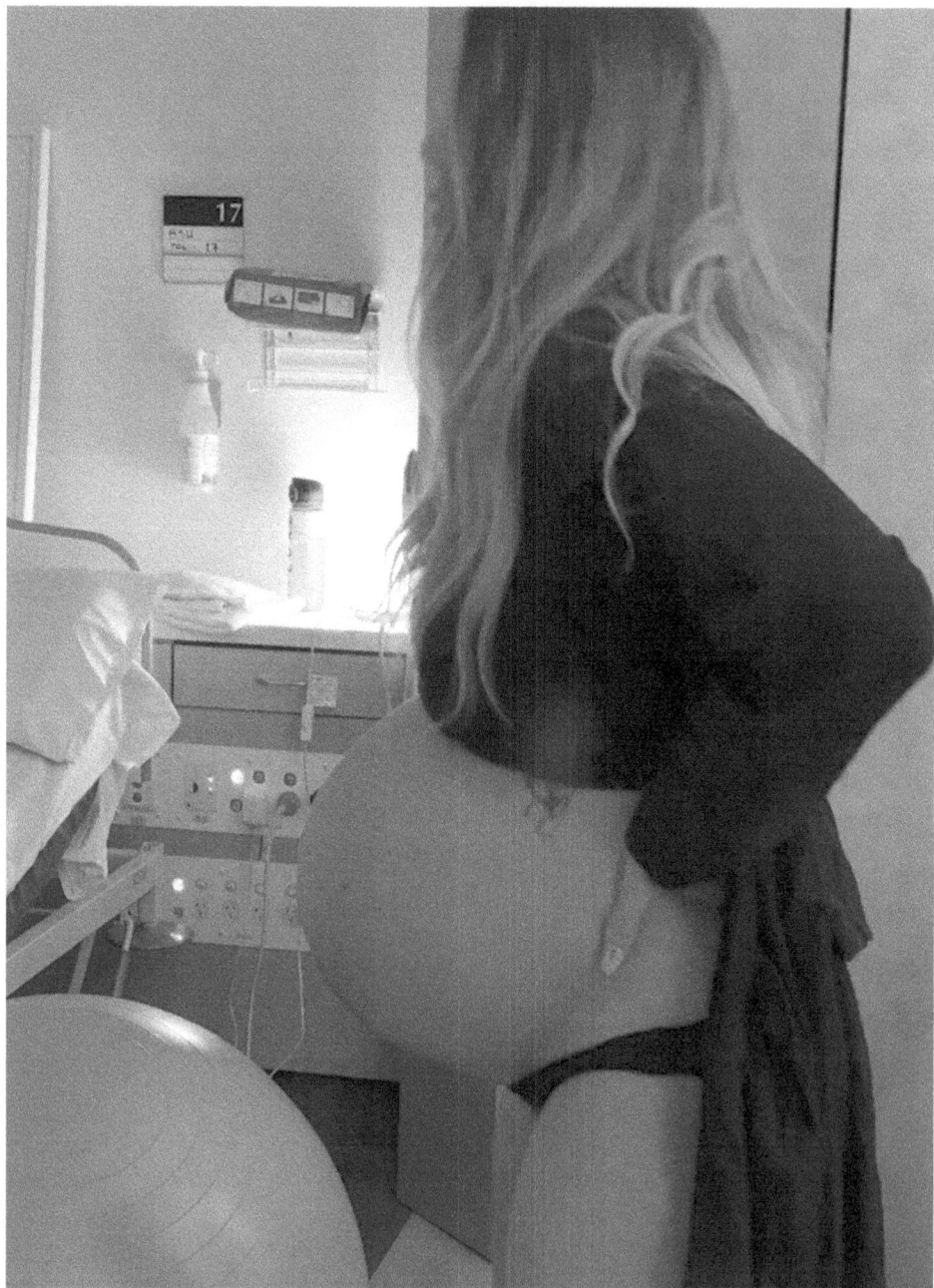

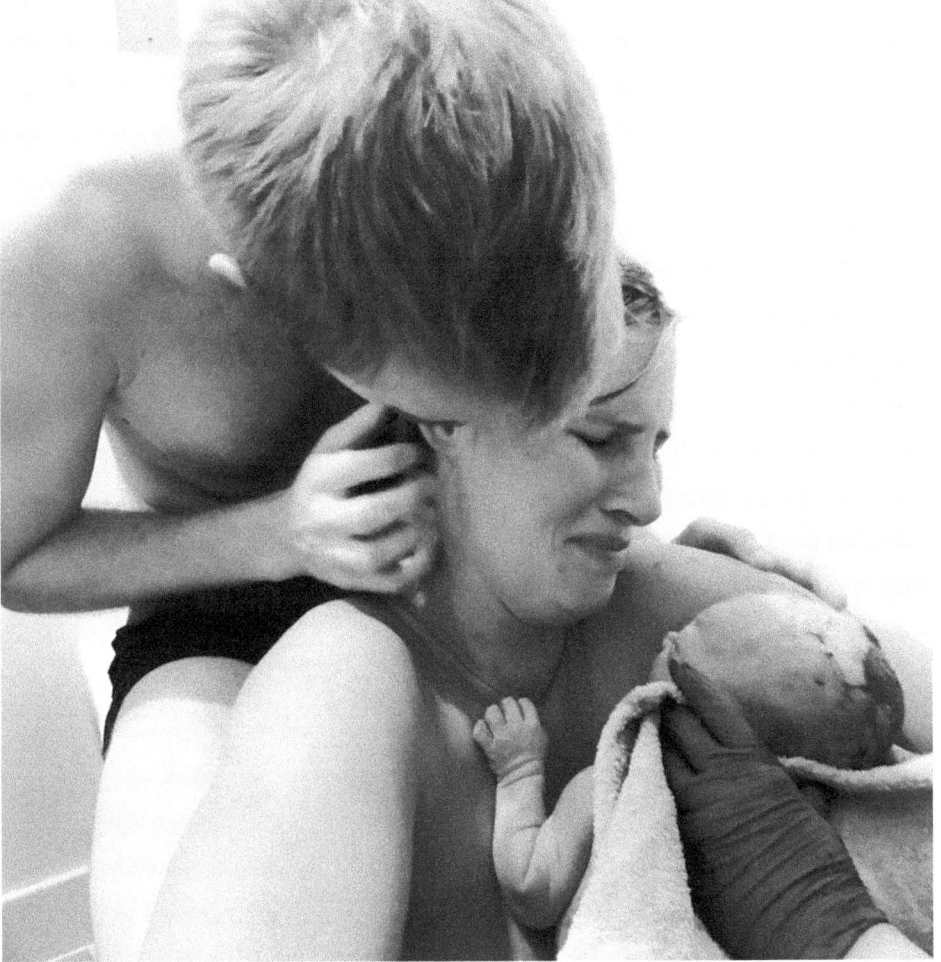

Midwife Crisis

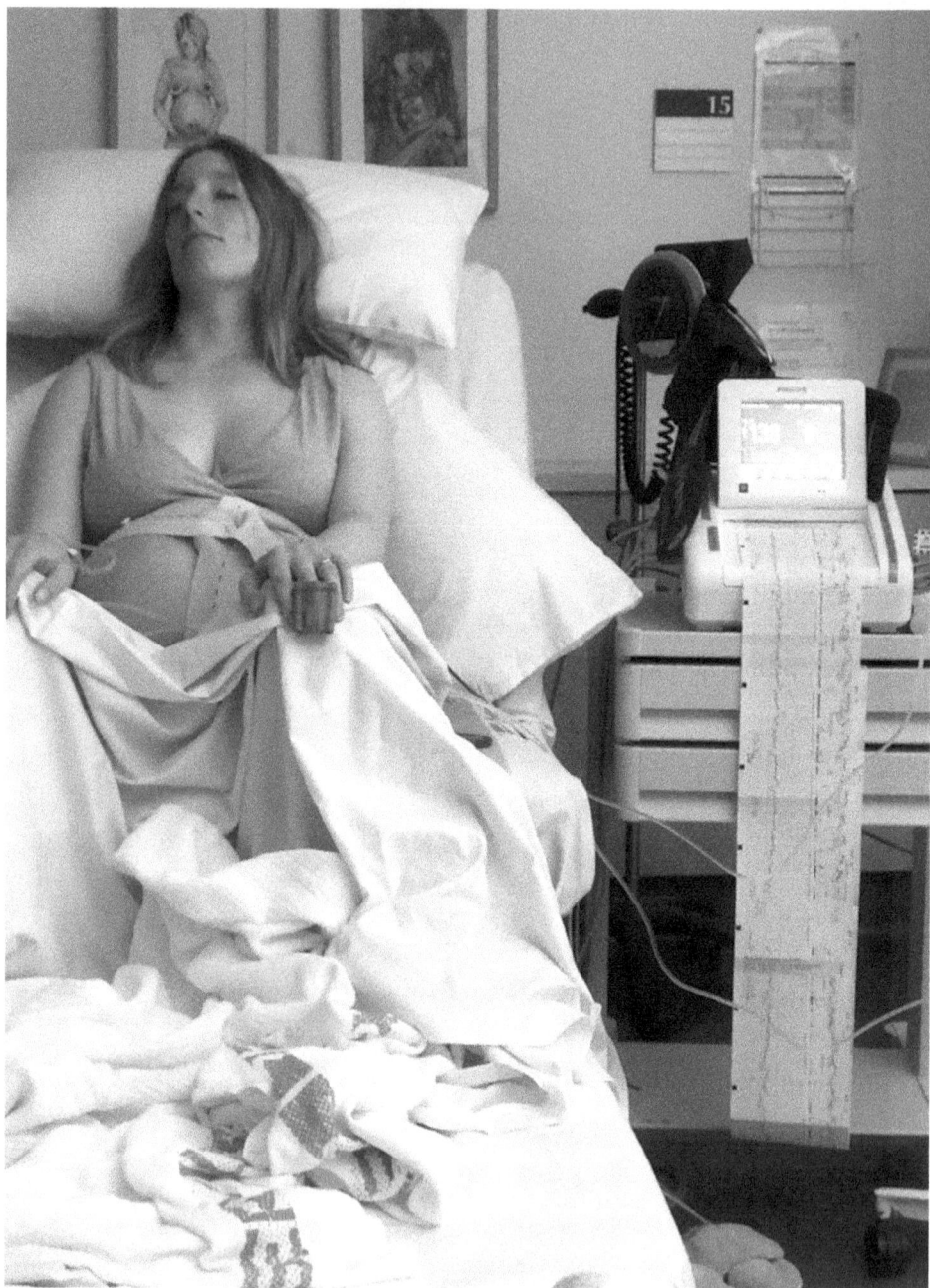

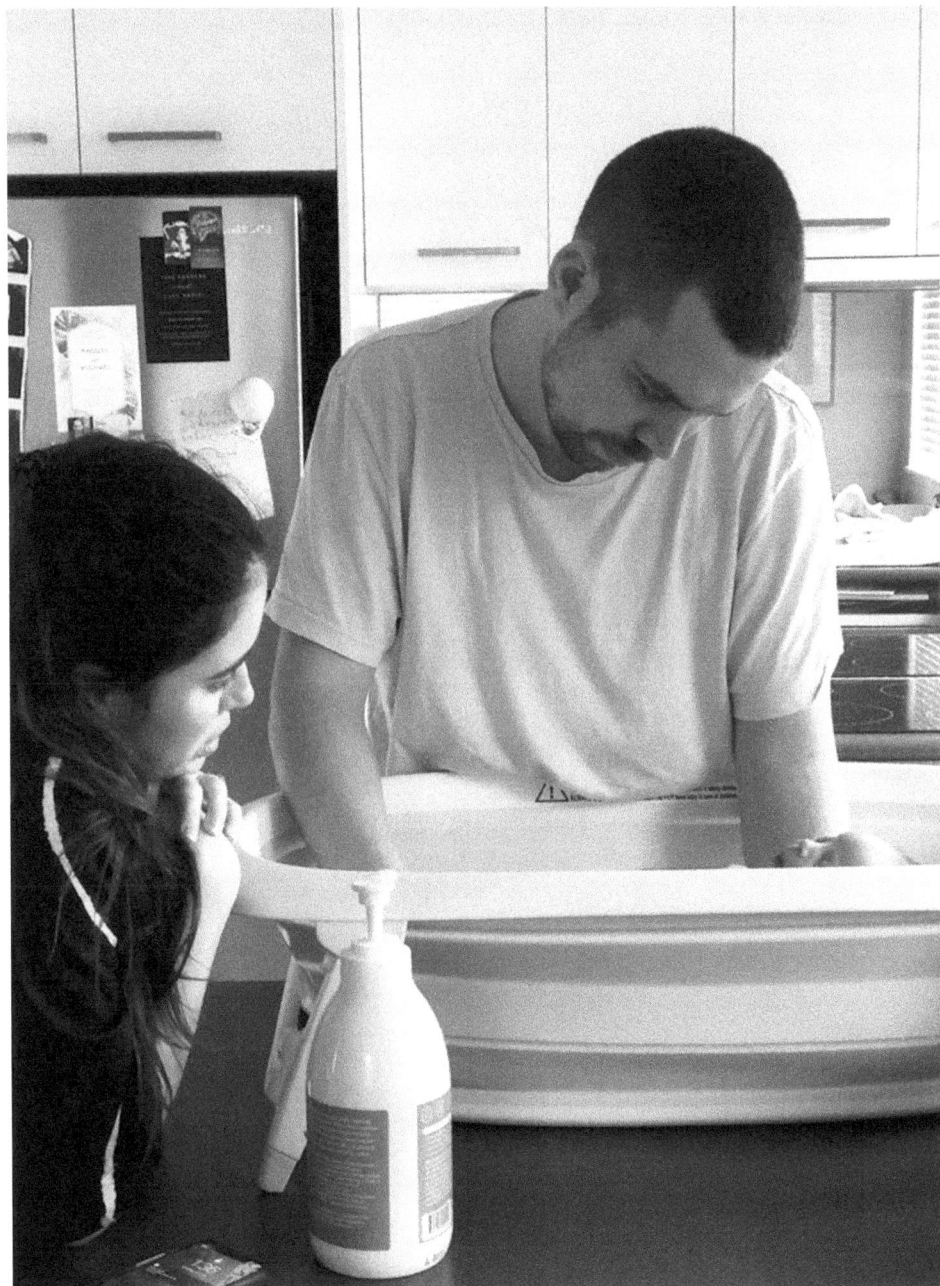

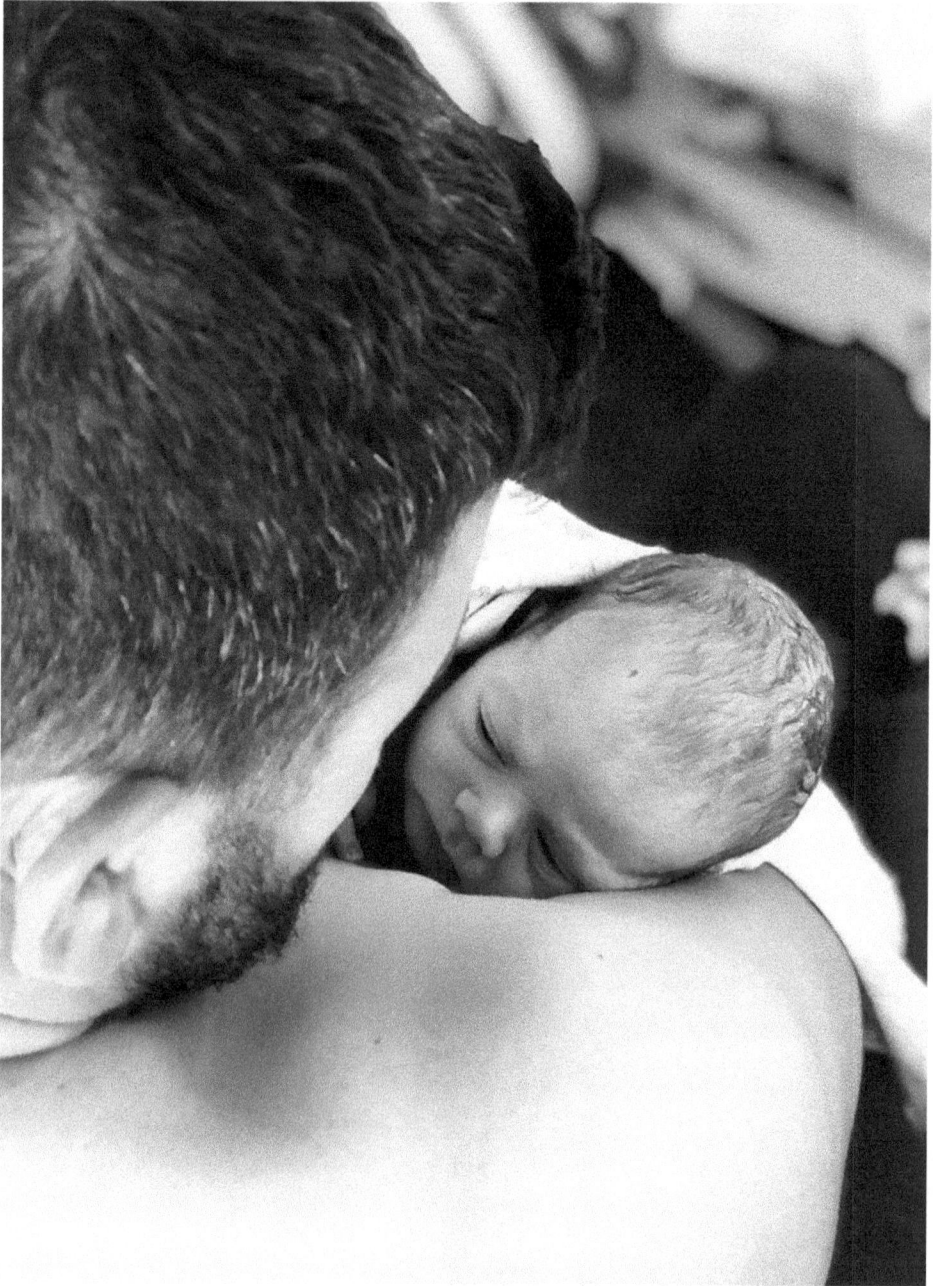

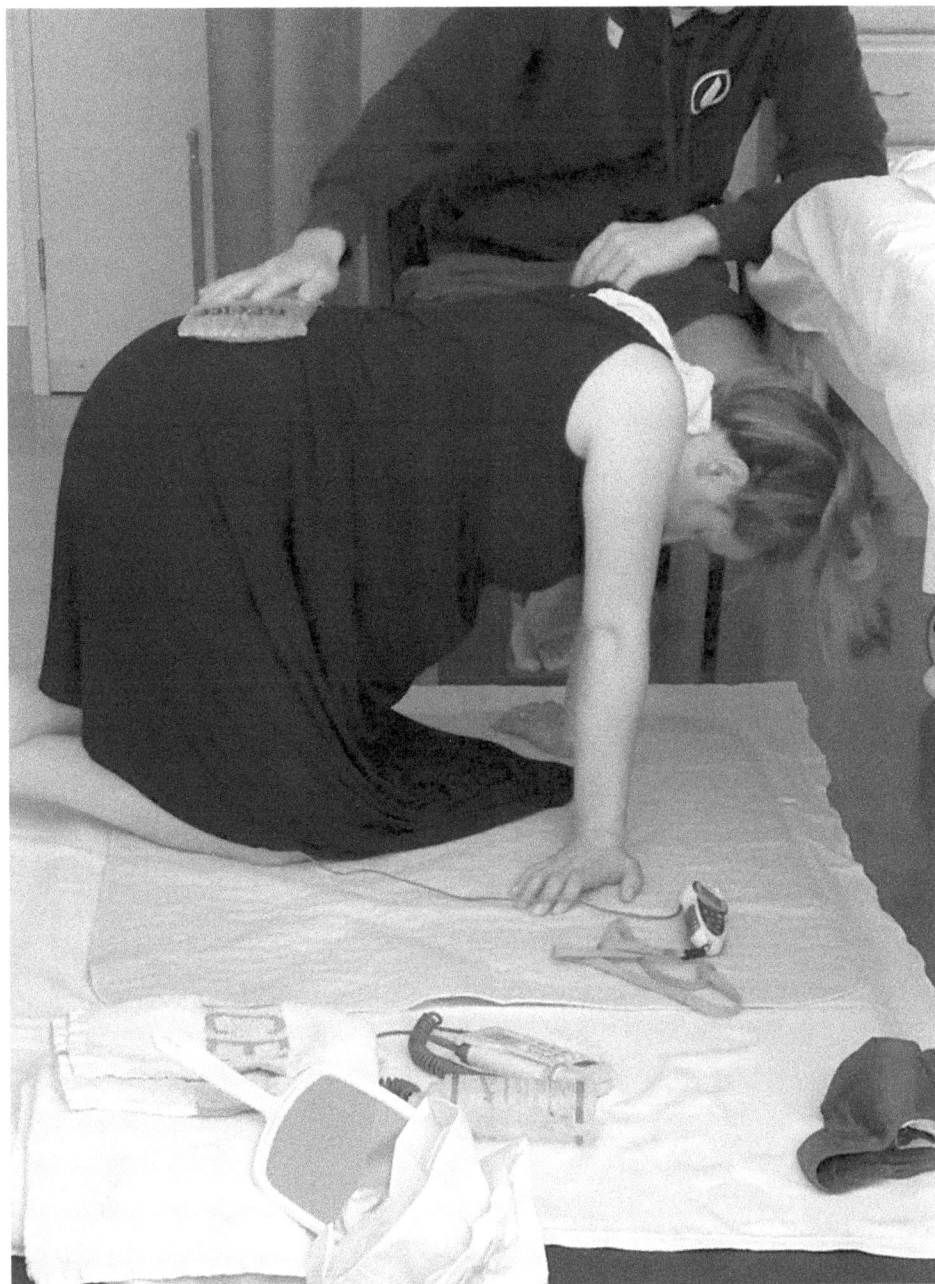

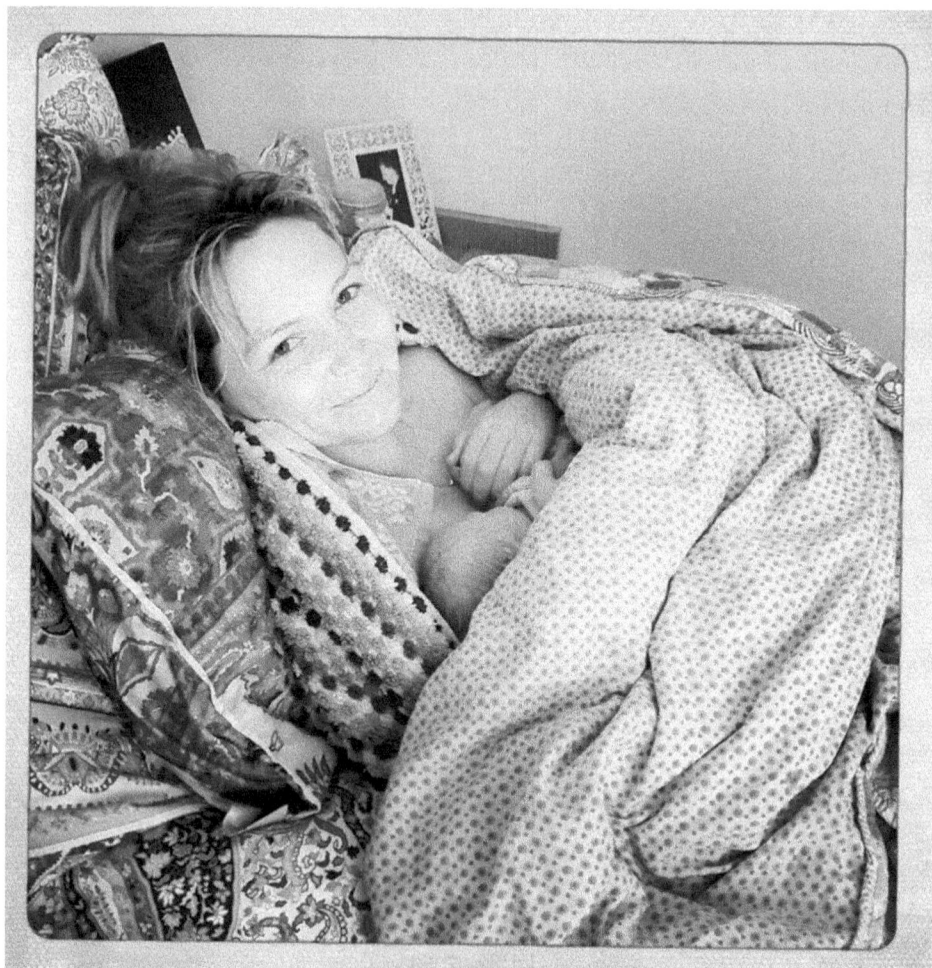

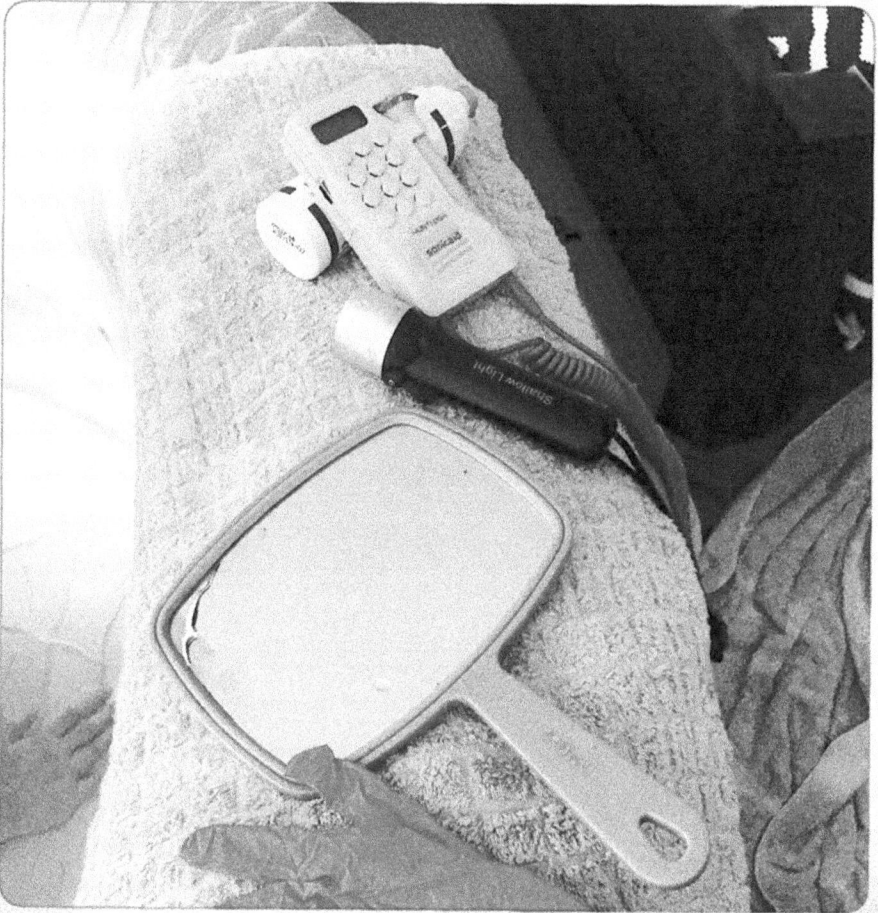

Midwife Crisis

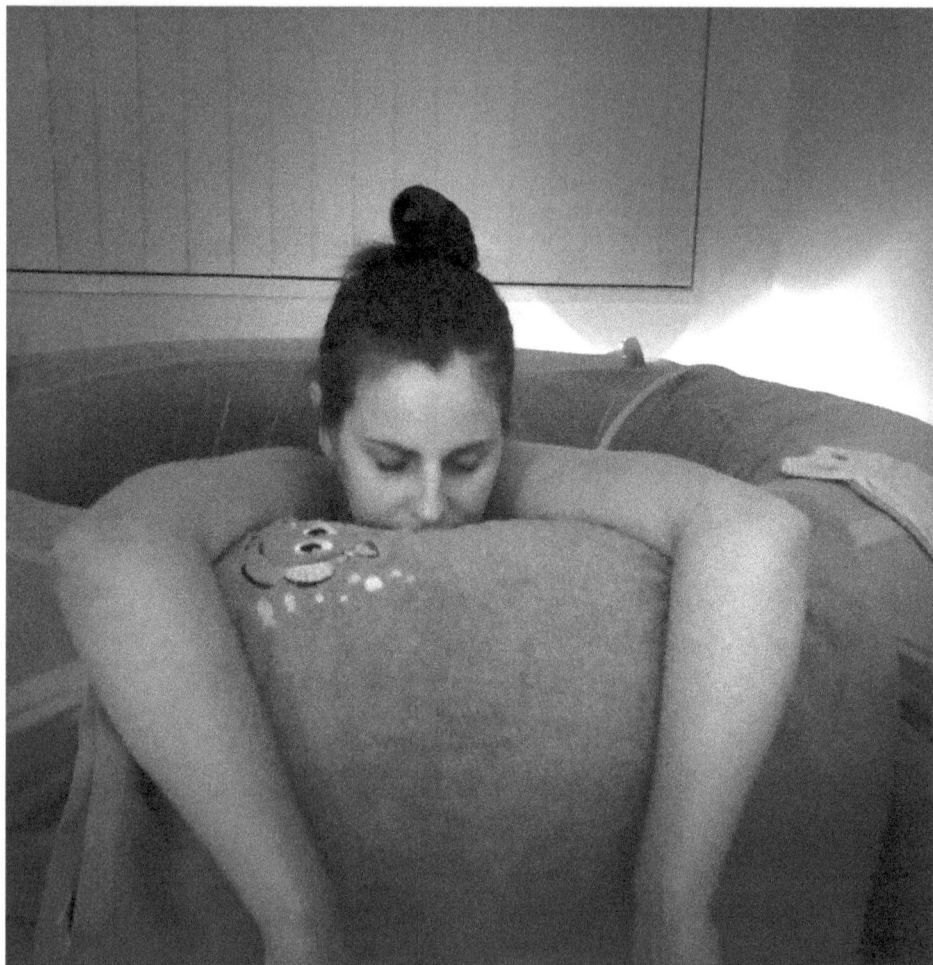

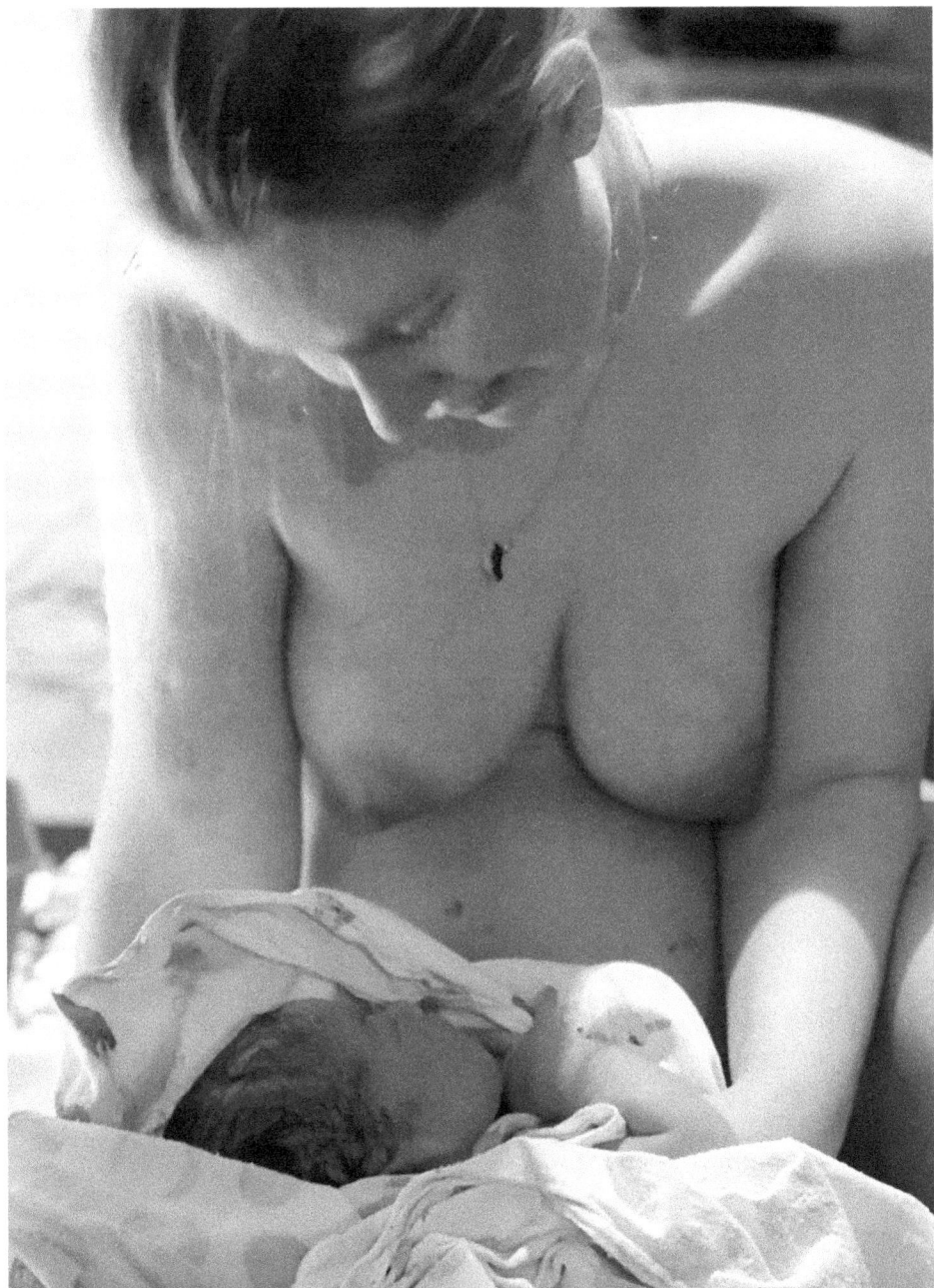

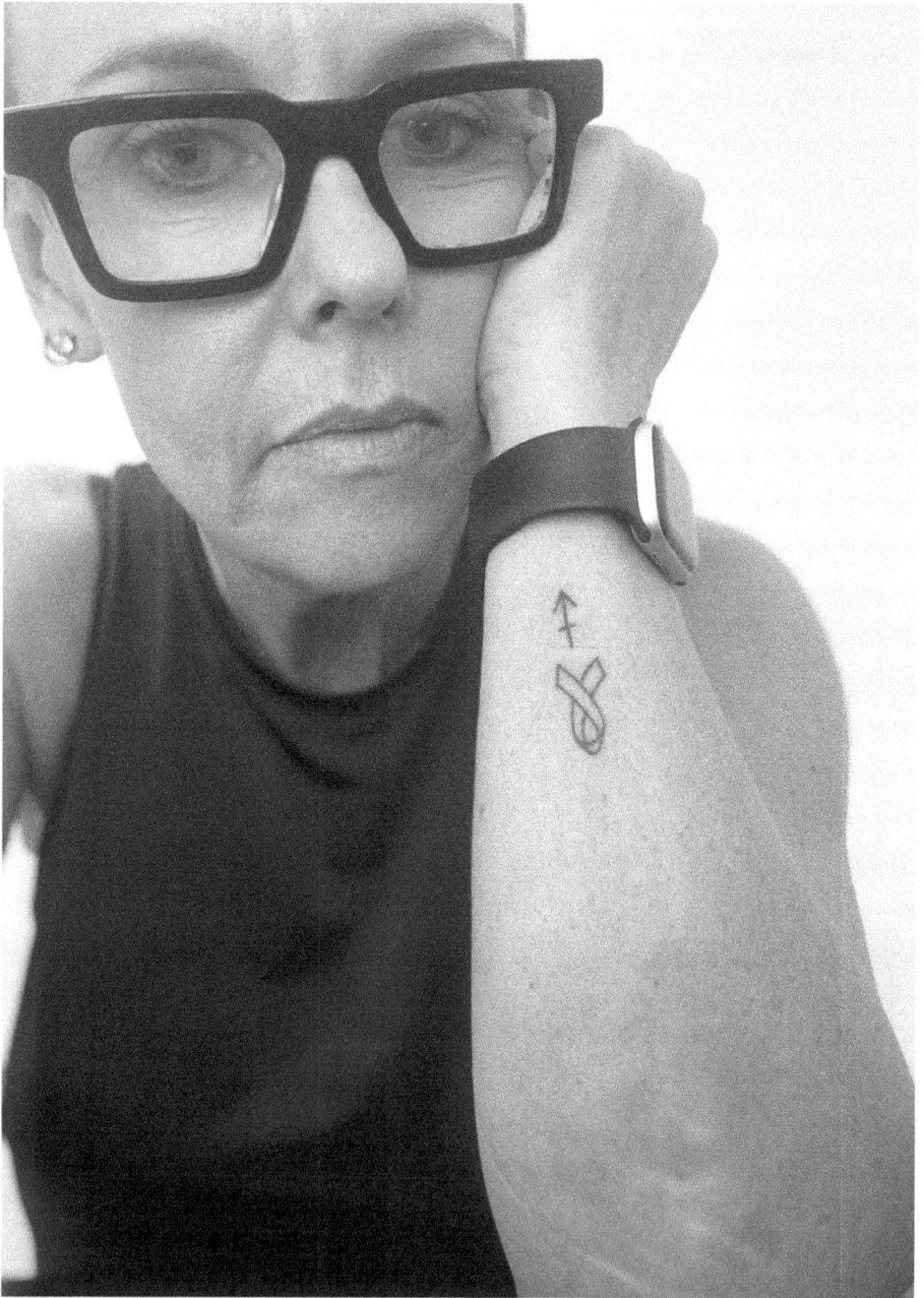

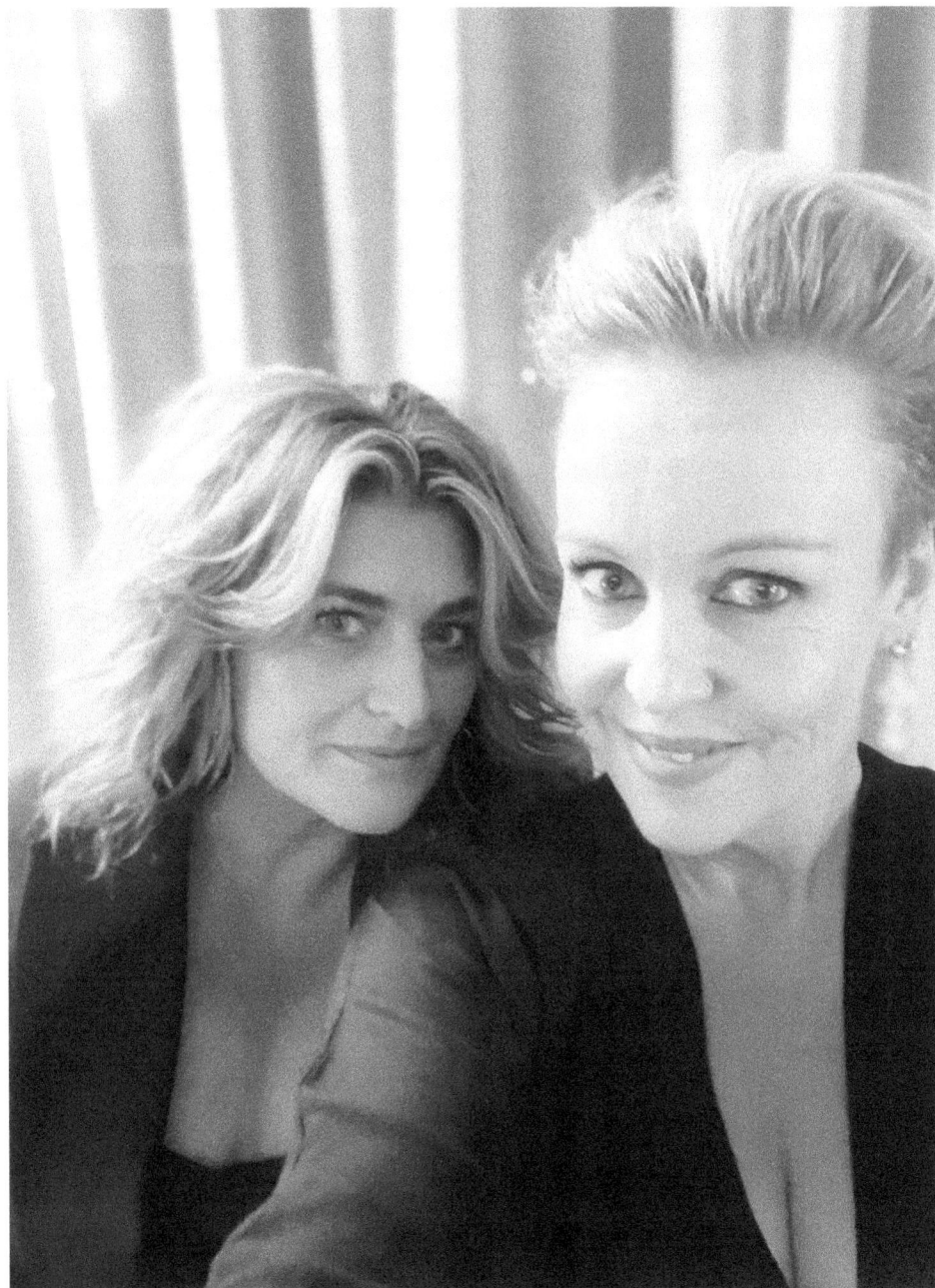

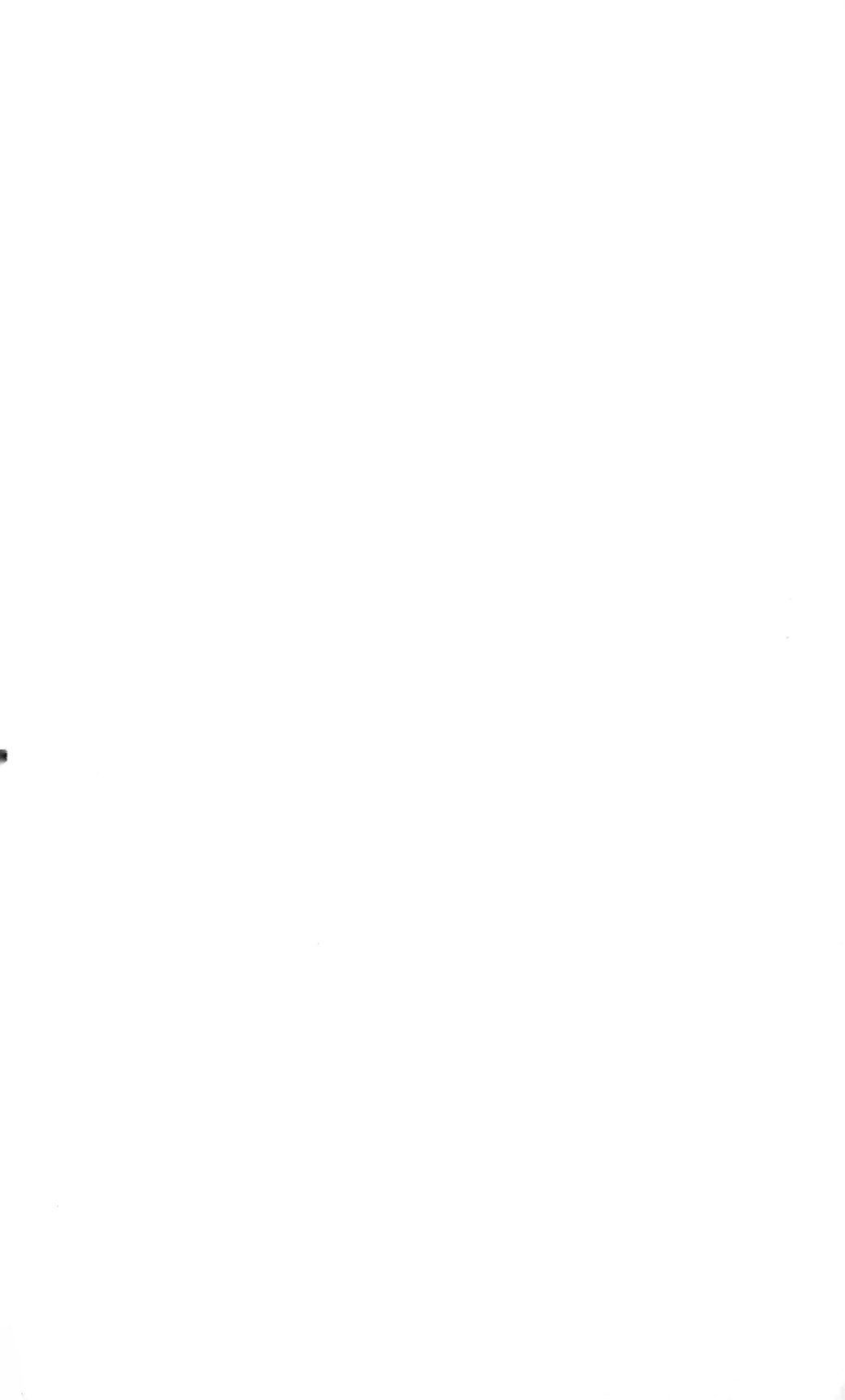

9 781923 255289